The Mainstreaming of Complementary and Alternative Medicine

Complementary and alternative medicine (CAM) is a major component of healthcare in most late modern societies. While there is increasing recognition of the need for more research in this area, it is frequently argued that such research should be directed towards establishing 'evidence' that will provide 'answers' to policy questions. However, complementary medicine is also a topic worthy of study in its own right, a historically contingent social product, and it is this sociological agenda that underpins *The Mainstreaming of Complementary and Alternative Medicine*.

Contributors to the book come from the UK, USA, Canada, Australia and New Zealand. They draw on their own research to explore issues such as the role of consumers as activists; the rhetoric of individual responsibility; the significance of evidence-based medicine; and contested boundaries in the workplace. The book also discusses specific processes relating to CAM practitioners, GPs and nurses.

Stepping back from the immediate demands of policy-making, *The Mainstreaming of Complementary and Alternative Medicine* allows a complex and informative picture to emerge of the different social forces at play in the integration of CAM with orthodox medicine. Complementing books that focus solely on practice, it will be relevant reading for all students following health sociology, health studies or healthcare courses, for medical students and medical and healthcare professionals, as well as academic CAM specialists.

Philip Tovey is Principal Research Fellow, School of Healthcare Studies, University of Leeds. **Gary Easthope** is Reader in Sociology, School of Sociology and Social Work, University of Tasmania. **Jon Adams** is Lecturer in Health Social Science, School of Medical Practice and Population Health, University of Newcastle, Australia.

D0006625

The Mainstreaming of Complementary and Alternative Medicine

Studies in Social Context

Edited by Philip Tovey,
Gary Easthope and Jon Adams

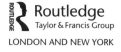

Routledge
Taylor & Francis Group

LONDON AND NEW YORK

First published 2004
by Routledge
11 New Fetter Lane, London EC4P 4EE

Simultaneously published in the USA and Canada
by Routledge
29 West 35th Street, New York, NY 10001

Routledge is an imprint of the Taylor & Francis Group

© 2004 Compilation and editorial material Philip Tovey,
Gary Easthope and Jon Adams; individual contributions,
the contributors

Typeset in Sabon and Gill by BC Typesetting, Bristol
Printed and bound in Great Britain by
The Cromwell Press, Trowbridge, Wiltshire

British Library Cataloguing in Publication Data
A catalogue record for this book is available from the British Library

Library of Congress Cataloging in Publication Data
A catalog record has been requested

ISBN 0–415–26700–5 (pbk)
ISBN 0–415–26699–8 (hbk)

For
Passenger N - LA, FB
Annie and Frank; Sallie and Bill

Contents

PART III
Boundary contestation in the workplace

Illustrations

Tables

Box

Notes on contributors

Jon Adams is a Lecturer in Health Social Science and co-ordinator of the qualitative research laboratory at the Centre for Clinical Epidemiology and Biostatistics, University of Newcastle, Australia. His main research interest is the sociology of CAM and he is currently researching CAM consumption and provision in Australia and Europe.

Heather Boon is an Assistant Professor in the Faculty of Pharmacy, University of Toronto, Canada. In addition, she is cross-appointed to the Department of Family and Community Medicine and the Department of Health Policy, Management and Evaluation, Faculty of Medicine, University of Toronto. Heather has founded the Toronto Complementary and Alternative Medicine Research Network. Her primary research interests are patients' use of complementary/alternative medicine, the safety and efficacy of natural health products, and complementary/alternative medicine regulation and policy issues.

Fran Collyer is a Lecturer in Sociology at the University of Sydney, Australia. Fran's research interests concern both the fields of sociology and social policy, and include the privatisation of public assets (particularly with regard to healthcare services); health financing and healthcare systems in Europe, Australia, the USA and Asia; the changing relationship between the nation state and the market; and science, technology and innovation.

Ian Coulter is a Professor in the School of Dentistry, University of California, Los Angeles, a Research Professor at Southern California University of Health Sciences, and a senior Health Consultant at RAND, USA. He is the Principal Investigator (PI) of the Evidence-Based Practice Center for Complementary and Alternative Medicine at RAND, and is the PI on a case study of integrative medicine.

Kevin Dew is a Senior Lecturer in Social Science and Health at the Department of Public Health, Wellington School of Medicine and Health

Sciences, University of Otago, New Zealand. His research interests include CAM, occupational health and health services research.

Gary Easthope is a Reader in Sociology at the University of Tasmania, Australia. He has taught at universities in England, Ireland, Canada and the USA. He has written on education, drug use, youth, environmental movements and research methods in addition to CAM, and is currently researching heritage sailing ships, as well as CAM use amongst Australian women.

Melinda Goldner is an Assistant Professor of Sociology at Union College in Schenectady, New York, USA. She has studied various aspects of the complementary and alternative medicine movement, including who is more likely to participate, how activists have changed their goals, and how physicians have responded to the movement.

Kahryn Hughes is a Senior Research Fellow at the Nuffield Institute for Health, University of Leeds, UK. Her main research interests include processes of identity formation in: negotiations of definitions of care, particularly in nursing; the sociology of complementary therapies; HIV/AIDS and anorexia nervosa; and women's networks in the context of community formation.

Merrijoy Kelner is a Professor Emeritus at the Institute for Human Development, Life Course and Aging at the University of Toronto, Canada. She leads a team of researchers in the area of CAM. Her research focuses on the ways in which several CAM groups are trying to gain a foothold in mainstream healthcare.

Philip Tovey is a Principal Research Fellow, School of Healthcare Studies, University of Leeds, UK. He has researched widely in the sociology of education and the sociology of health, and has published on CAM in a range of major international journals. He currently leads a CAM research programme that has a particular focus on cancer, and on developing a critical sociology of CAM and nursing.

Bryan S. Turner is Professor of Sociology at the University of Cambridge, UK. He has a long-standing interest in health sociology and is the author of *Medical Power and Social Knowledge* and *The Body and Society*. He is also, with Mike Featherstone, the founding editor of the journal *Body and Society*. He has also been concerned to develop the sociology of citizenship and human rights.

Beverley Wellman is a Medical Sociologist at the Institute for Human Development, Life Course and Aging at the University of Toronto, Canada. Her research focuses on complementary and alternative medicine with a special interest in the relationship between social networks, social capital and professionalisation.

Sandy Welsh is an Associate Professor of Sociology at the Unversity of Toronto, Canada. Her current areas of research include the professions, neighbourhood effects on health outcomes and sexual harassment. In addition to her work in the area of complementary and alternative medicine professions, she is a leading expert on sexual harassment in Canada.

Kevin White is a Reader in Sociology in the School of Social Sciences at the Australian National University. He has held appointments at Flinders University of South Australia, Wollongong University and Victoria University, Wellington, New Zealand. His research interests are in the sociology of health and illness, the historical sociology of health, and patterns of inequality in health.

Evan Willis is Professor of Sociology and Head of the Faculty of Humanities and Social Sciences on the Albury-Wodonga (regional) campus of La Trobe University. For most of his career he has been interested in the question of how illness mediates social relations and this has led him to an interest in complementary and alternative medicine, amongst other themes.

Foreword

The end(s) of scientific medicine?

Bryan S. Turner

The Mainstreaming of Complementary and Alternative Medicine (CAM) is a timely and challenging sociological account of the development and significance of complementary and alternative forms of medical therapeutics. These essays raise important questions about the medical profession and its clients, about the scientific claims of 'evidenced-based medicine' (EBM), and about the impact of modern (and possibly postmodern) consumer demand on healthcare and patient expectations. We need to understand these sociological investigations against the historical backdrop of the development of scientific, allopathic medicine and the consolidation of medical dominance, the early erosion of alternative systems of care, and their slow but steady revival so that what used to be the dubious practice of 'alternative medicine' eventually became 'complementary medicine' and more recently 'integrated medicine' or 'holistic medicine'. One important and problematic question is whether the growing acceptance of CAM is mainstreaming, co-opting or neutralising. What is evident, however, is that the growth of CAM represents a major transformation of the relationship between doctors and their patients, and between doctors and the larger scientific community.

The consolidation of professional scientific medicine in England was a late product of Victorian legislation and science (Porter 2001). Before 1858, physicians constituted a fluid and heterogeneous collection of learned men competing for clientele in an unregulated market. The reconstruction of the profession was achieved when the Medical Act of 1858 established a single Medical Register under the auspices of a General Medical Council. The Act united the doctors against their rivals – homeopaths, midwives, bonesetters, herbalists and itinerants. While the Act created a coherent profession, general practitioners remained underpaid and overworked, forced to be civil to their socially superior patients and to tolerate slow payments and bad debts. The general practitioner became an idealised figure – educated, long-suffering, poor, and the servant of the community.

In North America, the age of scientific medical training was launched by Flexner's (1910) report on *Medical Education in the United States and*

Canada. He argued that medical education had to be based on experimental science and laboratory instruction, and that medical schools should be part of a research university. He also made recommendations about entry requirements and the length of student education. The majority of existing medical schools failed to match his criteria and forty-six closed, including those educating women and the black community. His scientific assumptions also resulted in the decline of homoepathic training and provision. Partly through constraints on the supply of doctors, the Flexner reforms increased the status and pay of those doctors who came through the revised curriculum.

From 1910 to 1970 scientific medicine enjoyed a golden age of increasing influence, status and wealth. Research hospitals were models of scientific application, acute diseases were being eliminated, and the medical profession enjoyed the trust and respect of middle-class society. Flexner's assumptions laid the foundation for the medical model of illness, established the social conditions for medical dominance and produced the professional circumstances that underpinned the sick role (Parsons 1951). The doctor's clinical authority was unchallenged and the patient was expected to be docile and compliant. The American Medical Association (AMA) and the British Medical Association (BMA) were powerful professional lobbies that exercised significant political power on behalf of medical science, through Congress and Parliament respectively. The profession had considerable success in claiming that collectivist innovations in the delivery of healthcare would undermine the principles of individualism, self-help and self-reliance, upon which Western medicine had been built.

The end of the 'golden age of doctoring' (McKinlay and Marceau 1998) was signalled by Nixon's 1970 speech announcing a crisis in healthcare in the US: a crisis manifest in the rising numbers of uninsured Americans, the inability of germ theory to contribute to the treatment of chronic illnesses and major illnesses such as cancer and heart disease, the increasing use of alternative medicine and the growth of self-help movements.

Patient rights and consumer demand have pressured healthcare professionals to provide more holistic care. The slow but significant growth of healthcare insurance for CAM in the United states and the growing number of young doctors who do not join the AMA are regarded by some sociologists as indicative of an erosion of medical dominance (Pescosolido and Boyer 2001: 183). The medical profession has also changed under the impact of technical advances in medicine and commercial transformations of medical practice (Starr 1982). We can understand these changes within the framework of the sociology of the professions. Freidson (1970) in *Profession of Medicine* argued that the success of the medical profession rested not only on its political power but also on the trust of the public. These two dimensions of professionalism are medical dominance and the consulting ethic, in which the first requires state support, and the second depends on public confidence. Both have been transformed by the growth of corporate and global medical systems. These global changes are transforming the traditional doctor–patient relationship but they are also opening up new possibilities, the future directions of which are unclear.

In terms of public trust in the medical profession, technical inventions and discoveries of nineteenth-century medicine such as immunisation established the scientific authority of medicine as a profession. For the lay public, improvements in survival rates from surgery have been especially visible evidence of the scientific basis of contemporary medical practice. Although the quality of general practice still depends in large measure on inter-personal skills that can only be fully acquired through experience rather than training, the status of medical institutions in society depends significantly on 'hard' science and technology. Medical technology presents simultaneously and paradoxically the promise of significant therapeutic improvements in the management of illness, and significant risks to the well-being and comfort of patients. This tension between the art of healing and the science of disease is part of what Gadamer (1996) has called the modern 'enigma of health'.

Professional medicine has long been concerned to regulate, largely un-successfully, self-medication and 'folk medicine' (Bakx 1991), but it is also important to control scientific medicine. In order to gain the benefits of medical innovation, there has to be some regulation of the social and cultural risks associated with contemporary medical sciences, for example in relation to cloning, new reproductive technologies, organ transplants, surgical intervention for fetal abnormalities, cosmetic surgery, the prescription of antidepressants, cryonically frozen patients or sex selection of children. Who should exercise these regulatory constraints or governance over the medical sciences? The professions and governments are no longer able to deliver effective oversight, because the globalisation of markets makes legislative and political regulation problematic (Kass 2002). The result is an endless political cycle of risk, audit, regulation and deregulation. This cycle of political confrontations and compromises with the scientific establishment inflames lay suspicion of expert opinion and erodes the relation of trust between patients and doctors. In Britain, the BMA has been criticised for its failure to monitor effectively doctors who have been charged with criminal offences or malpractice. The nadir of trust in doctor–patient relations in Britain in recent history may have been finally reached by the revelations about Dr Shipman who, in the latter part of his career, killed hundreds of elderly patients in his care. The apparent instability and contradictions in the expert advice surrounding the foot and mouth epidemic of 2001 in Britain further eroded the authority of scientific opinion. Lay confidence in science and the food chain has been further battered by a 20 to 30 per cent rise in Creutzfeld-Jakob disease in

Britain. These examples suggest that the tensions between public trust, uninsurable risk and scientific legitimacy have generally undermined confidence in expert systems (Giddens 1990; Beck 1992) and, as a result, the public has experimented with alternative and less intrusive healing systems.

Any sociological understanding of medicine in contemporary society must examine the economics of the corporate structure of medical practice and has to locate that structure within a framework of global commercial and cultural processes. The deregulation of global markets has had the unintended consequence of bringing about the globalisation of disease. For example, the return of the 'old' infectious diseases (TB, malaria, typhoid and cholera) will have significant negative consequences for the economies of the developing world, but they will also reappear in the affluent West as a consequence of the globalisation of transport, tourism and labour markets. It is unlikely that corporations will adopt policies of corporate citizenship sufficiently quickly or effectively to exercise constraint and to institutionalise environmental audits to regulate their impact on local communities. However, these global developments have also created new opportunities for the exercise of consumer power as a mechanism whereby the negative impact of corporate enterprise on fragile communities and environments can be challenged. Future developments of healthcare must be connected with debates about civil society and human rights. We need to realise that health – more even than employment, education and welfare – is the fundamental entitlement of citizenship, but this entitlement is often difficult to implement within a world economy where risks are global. The question of health as entitlement raises difficult political and policy questions, because there is an inevitable tension between citizenship as a bundle of national rights and obligations, and human rights as a system of entitlement that does not rest directly on the sovereignty of particular nation states.

I have already indicated that the model of the professional doctor that shaped Parsons' approach to the professions is now obsolete with the passing of the golden age of medicine. The growth of corporate control over medical care has contributed to the decline of professional autonomy, initiative and social status. The neo-liberal emphasis on the free market and aggressive entrepreneurship has brought about a decline in the social status of general practitioners by converting many into the hired employees of profit-making, private-sector health systems. Furthermore, the contemporary development of healthcare in the US has brought about a new emphasis on medical specialisation that has undermined, or at least threatened, the occupational coherence and solidarity of medicine as a professional group. In addition to this internal division, with the growth of consumer groups and with malpractice legislation and public alarm with technological medicine, there has been a renewed interest in more holistic medical services through alternative and complementary systems. The commercialisation of medicine and the dominance of free-market principles have had the paradoxical consequence of eroding the foundations of the traditionally autonomous professional physician as an individual provider of care in a direct relationship to the client.

While neo-liberal policies may have changed the conditions under which the traditional autonomy of the medical profession was sustained, these policies have also had serious consequences for consumers. For example, in the USA poverty has increased by 30 per cent among children since 1979; between 1981 and 1982, eleven states showed increases in the infant mortality rate and also showed considerable differences between black and white mortality rates. These rising infant mortality rates are associated with an increase in poverty and unemployment, a decline in nutrition and the loss of health insurance coverage through the new limitations on Medicaid. During the same period, the private health sector has enjoyed buoyant profitability and expansion. The economic and political importance of the tax cuts under the Reagan administration was that, by reducing revenue to the state, they curtailed the ability of future governments to introduce new social welfare programmes to remove hardship, stimulate employment and restore welfare measures. As medicine has become increasingly specialised, the general practitioner has become the conduit into medical care through whom the patient is referred to specialists further down the chain of delivery. The traditional relations of trust that characterised medical practice have been eroded by the commercialisation of services and the increasing anonymity of medical practitioners in relation to patients. Patients have turned to self-help partly because they cannot afford allopathic medicine and partly because they distrust invasive medication and treatment.

The development of new reproductive technologies, genetic engineering and the enhancement of human traits points towards a 'second medical revolution' that combines microbiology and informational science. This revolution presents a major challenge to traditional institutions and religious cosmologies, but it may also present a threat to the processes of political governance. The notion of risk society provokes questions about the unintended consequences of medical change, about whether the technological imperative can be regulated, and about the relationships between pure research, commercialisation and academic autonomy. For example, pharmaceutical companies have turned to contract research organisations (CROs) rather than universities to undertake basic research on drugs. These CROs are cheaper and also less independent than academic institutions. The academic community has argued that such research is not systematically published and is unlikely to be critical of the pharmaceutical products. In short, such 'private' research is not compatible with the public norms of publication, debate and criticism that are assumed to be essential to scientific objectivity.

Medical institutions and professions are subject to global pressures, especially from competitive insurance and funding arrangements. To take one obvious illustration, the ownership of the pharmaceutical industry is global and dominated by a limited number of corporations – ICI, Ciba and Hoetchst – which presents serious problems with respect to the regulation of the industry, the freedom of market relations and medical practice. We are also on the verge of healthcare systems that will depend on global electronic communications. One remarkable example is 'telesurgery' that involves the use of robot-assisted distance surgery. These techniques pioneered by the US military in order to provide expert medical services in the field could also make a valuable contribution to aid workers in developing societies and provide important training services for young surgeons. It is assumed that in the future patients and doctors will use broadband technologies to deliver healthcare packages to homes and hospitals. The growth of e-health will create virtual hospitals, transform health education, deliver health services to elderly or disabled patients who have limited mobility, and improve health delivery to remote rural communities. The technology and delivery systems for such innovations will be necessarily global, and it will be organised and owned by global health corporations.

Although the dominant trend of much recent medical sociology has been to emphasise the negative effects of globalisation and to regard e-health as a further commodification of medicine, there are alternative trends that indicate a growth in consumer autonomy, increased involvement of patient groups in decision-making and an erosion of medical dominance in favour of 'bottom-up' participation. For a variety of specific conditions and diseases, there has been increased use by patients of websites for care, support and information. The model of the consumer/patient lobby group was provided by the HIV/AIDS epidemic, where activists have successfully challenged medical control and shaped the nature of AIDS research and research funding. AIDS websites played an important part in organising such movements (Altman 2001). Another particularly good example is cystic fibrosis (CF). As life expectancy rates for sufferers have increased to around thirty years of age, public health-care systems have had to rely increasingly on home help and lay caregivers. There is now a range of CF websites that provide health information such as on the use of intravenous injections for home care. The result is to sideline professional medical control and to transform the nature of medical authority. With the increase in chronic illness as a result of HIV/AIDS, ageing and changes in lifestyle, the management of care may pass more and more into lay hands with the support of e-health systems. Obviously this is a mixed blessing as more care is devolved to female heads of households, but it does represent also an increase in lay power. Of course, corporate e-health will take a predatory interest in 'nativistic' or 'indigenous pharmacy', will seek to commercialise alternative healthcare and to monopolise medical knowledge and research.

We may envisage an endlessly circular struggle between centralised and localised e-health, and between corporate and lay interests. The growth of CAM will clearly be assisted by global information systems that work at a local level, because patients will be directly selecting health-care alternatives from websites.

This collection of essays raises, as I have indicated here, acute issues relating to the relation between scientific knowledge and power. This theme in contemporary medical sociology arose in response to the influence of Foucault (1973) whose historical work on the birth of the clinic demonstrated the intimate connections between the French Revolution, the growth of anatomy and the transformation of the concept of disease. Today we are going through a revolution of equal magnitude. The twentieth-century monopoly of mainstream healthcare and provision that was enjoyed by professional medicine and the dominance of allopathic science have both been undermined, but obviously not eroded, by a complex set of global processes: new technologies, changes in consumer demand, the globalisation of medical systems, the differentiation and fragmentation of scientific knowledge, the transformation of the pattern of disease and a variety of new social movements. New configurations of power are producing new systems of knowledge within which CAM will come to play an important, but probably unpredictable part. The global revolution in healthcare will in turn compel the scientific community to reconsider and redefine the ends of medicine.

References

Altman, D. (2001) *Global Sex*, Chicago and London: University of Chicago Press.

Bakx, K. (1991) 'The "eclipse" of folk medicine in Western society', *Sociology of Health and Illness* 13(1): 20–38.

Beck, U. (1992) *Risk Society: towards a new modernity*, London: Sage.

Flexner, A. (1910) *Medical Education in the United states and Canada*, New York: Carnegie Foundation for the Advancement of Teaching.

Foucault, M. (1973) *The Birth of the Clinic*, London: Tavistock.

Freidson, E. (1970) *Profession of Medicine. A study of the sociology of applied knowledge*, New York: Harper and Row.

Gadamar, H-G. (1996) *The Enigma of Health. The art of healing in a scientific age*, Cambridge: Polity Press.

Giddens, A. (1990) *The Consequences of Modernity*, Cambridge: Polity Press.

Kass, L.R. (2002) *Life, Liberty and the Defense of Dignity. The challenge for bioethics*, San Francisco: Encounter Books.

McKinlay, J.D. and Marceau, L.D. (1998) 'The impact of managed care on patients' trust in medical care and their physicians'. Paper presented at the American Public Health Association, Washington DC, November (cited in W.A. Cockerham (ed.) (2001) *The Blackwell Companion to Medical Sociology*, Oxford: Blackwell, p. 196).

Parsons, T. (1951) *The Social System*, London: Routledge and Kegan Paul.

Pescosolido, B.A. and Boyer, C.A. (2001) 'The American health care system: entering the twenty-first century with high risk, major challenges and great opportunities', in W. Cockerham (ed.) *The Blackwell Companion to Medical Sociology*, Oxford: Blackwell, pp. 180–98.

Porter, R. (2001) *Bodies Politic. Disease, death and doctors in Britain 1650–1900*, London: Reaktion Books.

Starr, P. (1982) *The Social Transformation of American Medicine. The rise of a sovereign profession and the making of a vast industry*, New York: Basic Books.

Introduction

Philip Tovey, Gary Easthope and Jon Adams

Complementary and alternative medicine (CAM)[1] is now a major part of the healthcare system in all advanced societies.[2] It is also a common part of discourse in medicine and healthcare. This growth of interest has only partially been matched by academic study of it. Indeed, over recent years there has been an increasing recognition that CAM is essentially under-researched (House of Lords 2000). However, with this recognition has come an increasing concentration on a particular form of research – that geared towards the production of an evidence base and/or an immediate relevance to policy and practice.

These research priorities are reflected in much of the work that is published on CAM. In both standard medical journals and in CAM specific publications the emphasis is squarely on the problems of efficacy and of issues to do with practice, most recently integrative practice. Most books written in the field follow this pattern, being either concerned with the demonstrable value of individual therapies (Ernst *et al.* 2001) or being written as 'how to' guides geared towards practitioners (see, for example, Vickers 1993; Downey 1997; Tanvir 2001).

However, there is a different research agenda and a further set of writings on the subject – those that can be loosely grouped together as constituting a sociology of CAM. Here the emphases are rather different. While many of the topics may seem familiar from the policy driven agenda – regulation, the evidence base, use of CAM by general practitioners (GPs), nurses and others – they are treated in a very different way. Assumptions are challenged; motives and strategies are explored. CAM is first and foremost examined as a topic worthy of study in its own right, as a historically specific social product. Phenomena are studied in their social context. It is this sociological rather than policy-driven starting point that underpins this book. While the research covered herein may provide insights of practical benefits, that is not usually its fundamental purpose.

Central to this more in-depth sociological approach is the recognition that to merely seek to quantify effect, or to establish models of appropriate practice in tightly defined situations, is to only scratch the surface of the possibilities of an academic engagement with CAM. To understand the contemporary forms and contents of CAM there is a need to step back from the often hurriedly established demands of policy-makers, and to explicitly include in analyses reference to how the arena is marked by complexity and contingency, diversity and dispute and is in a state of constant change (Tovey and Adams 2001).

So, for instance, analyses need to start from a recognition that the growth of CAM in recent decades is historically contingent and that, like orthodox medicine, it is also a social product. Unlike orthodox medicine, however, a key aspect of that contingency is that it faced, as it developed, an already firmly entrenched medical orthodoxy supported by the state (Willis 1989).

Viewing CAM as a historically contingent and contested social product produces a very complex picture of a diverse field of therapies, products and relationships. Whilst we can note the existence of contestation between orthodox medicine and CAM, we should not fall back on the conventional picture that presents CAM versus orthodox medicine as the key to understanding CAM. Neither orthodox medicine nor CAM is a monolith. There are disputes and boundary claims being made both within orthodox medicine and within CAM. Not all medical practitioners agree on what constitutes orthodox medicine and not all CAM practitioners agree on what constitutes the alternative or the complementary (see Tovey and Adams 2001). In these disputes CAM can itself be used to assert boundaries within orthodox medicine, and make claims to particular skills or techniques, as, for example, in the case of nursing and therapeutic touch (see Trevelyan and Booth 1994). Similarly, within CAM some practitioners seek alliance with orthodox medicine, using orthodox medical courses as part of the training of their therapists (for example chiropractic). The term 'complementary', and more recently the term 'integrative' medicine, are signals of this complex social interaction.

Both orthodox medicine and CAM are constantly changing social products influenced by each other and by other social forces over which they have little or no control. The direction and pace of change is affected by the history of a particular region or country, so that homeopathy is popular among physicians in the UK, Germany, US and France (Wardwell 1994) and acupuncture among physicians in Australia (Easthope et al. 1998), while hydrotherapy is a major modality in Germany and herbal remedies are used both there and in China (Ullman 1993). Other contingencies such as changing state regulation affect which particular therapies are successful. For example, the Netherlands has recently allowed some modalities to receive limited state recognition and funding (Schepers and Hermans 1999) and the state of Victoria, in Australia, has legislated to register traditional Chinese medical practitioners (see Willis and White, Chapter 3). Less obviously, changing social structures in some countries or regions may create more middle-class consumers seeking preventive health measures through CAM.

Book structure and content

The aim of the book, then, is to bring together sociologically informed pieces about key issues in the ongoing mainstreaming of CAM. We have drawn together contributors from the UK, Australia, New Zealand, Canada and the US, many of whom base their arguments around empirical research conducted in those countries. An awareness of our principal concerns of complexity and contingency, social diversity, and change are evident across many of the chapters. However, we should be clear that our intention has not been to achieve a consensus – a single view about what constitutes *the* research priorities or *the* approach through which these should be studied. Authors have drawn on their own research agendas, theoretical preferences and empirical foci. That this may produce views that may at times conflict is welcomed in the spirit of open critical engagement with a relatively new area of social enquiry.

The book is divided into three parts: 'Consumption in Cultural Context', 'The Structural Context of the State and the Market' and 'Boundary Contestation in the Workplace'. These should not be seen to represent discrete areas of social life. The topics are, in practice, fundamentally interconnected: consumption is only possible in the presence of provision, that provision is influenced by political policy and so on. Moreover, there are other issues (inequalities and provision, group-based mediation of consumption, etc.) that relate to a full understanding of CAM in advanced societies but are not covered in this book.

Part 1, 'Consumption in Cultural Context', deals with the use or consumption of CAM. This is a wide-ranging theme. And this diversity is reflected in the very different emphases of the opening section's two chapters. In Chapter 1, Goldner draws on her empirical work in the USA to advance the case that the activity of CAM consumers (as consumers) creates a fluid social movement. This is a social movement without leaders or organisation and one driven by individual consumer choice in a society, the USA, in which consumption is a central defining feature. Each individual CAM user by using CAM techniques, by educating friends about CAM, and by agitating for changes in healthcare funding and institutions creates a social movement in support of CAM.

While we may be at the early stages of teasing out issues to do with the individual and collective identity in relation to consumption (or provision for that matter), one recurrent feature of contemporary health rhetoric that will need to be considered in such work is that relating to a personal responsibility for one's own health. In Chapter 2, Hughes picks up this issue and compares the way the patient/client is conceived in CAM and in the UK

National Health Service. She demonstrates that both see the individual as a consumer taking responsibility for their health. However, in CAM, taking responsibility is part of the actual process of healing whereas in the NHS it is manifested by making a choice between healers and/or by actions to reduce health risks. Thus, taking responsibility for one's health for those engaged in CAM treatments is continuous, while in the NHS it is episodic.

In each of the chapters of Part I, then, the importance of locating action in social context, and indeed of seeing that action as a transaction between, on the one hand, personal needs, wants and desires and, on the other, the possibilities, potential and limitations generated by that context, has been emphasised. Until we are able to draw on more focused empirical work, much of this notion of context will remain relatively abstract, as will the processes through which the joint production of CAM realities takes place.

In Part II, 'The Structural Context of the State and the Market', we turn to issues of context that are more immediately tangible: more directly identifiable as trends, policies and commercial realities that CAM practitioners and users must engage with, albeit on different levels and in different forms.

In Chapter 3, Willis and White tackle perhaps the core policy challenge – evidence-based medicine/practice (EBM): an issue that transcends any divide between orthodox and non-orthodox practice. In this chapter the authors look at the implications of evidence-based medicine for CAM. They argue that the 'gold standard' of EBM – the randomised control trial (RCT) – is usually not appropriate to CAM therapies, most of which assert the variability, and primacy, of the individual, making standardised treatments impossible. However, EBM by its emphasis on (clinical) outcomes rather than the (scientific) understanding of processes does mean that CAM therapies can be judged on the same criteria as more orthodox therapies. They go on to point out that success in proving the efficacy of certain therapeutic techniques or alternative medications may lead to their cooption by orthodox medicine. They conclude by demonstrating that the increasing acceptance of traditional Chinese medicine and naturopathy in Australia by the state owed nothing to EBM but rather was, as with chiropractic in New Zealand (described in Chapter 4), a result of clinical testimonies from consumers.

If questions relating to evidence are perhaps the high profile point of discussion, then regulation is not far behind. It is an issue that is bound up with the cornerstones of the historically grounded differentiation between orthodox and non-orthodox provision – power, legitimacy, inclusion/exclusion – and feeds into recurring discourses such as those built around 'quackery'. Dew (Chapter 4) examines a Royal Commission into Chiropractic in New Zealand, demonstrating how legitimation may be a two-edged sword. Chiropractors were able to gain recognition as a profession despite medical opposition because they were able to draw on the clinical legitimacy of testimonials from their clients. However, they only gained recognition from the state by limiting their claims and practice to dealing with back problems. Further, although the state recognised their right to practice independently of medicine and recommended that they should train doctors in dealing with back problems, in everyday practice nothing has changed. Doctors have not given them access to hospitals nor have they sought training from chiropractors.

In the case of both EBM and regulation we are primarily in the realm of the state, or at least of formal bodies ostensibly engaged in working towards maximising public good. However, there is another context that impacts on the CAM arena from a very different starting point, and is oriented towards goals that are based squarely within the commercial world. In Chapter 5, Collyer demonstrates that the marketplace has, over the heads of practitioners as it were, integrated CAM and orthodox medicine. Using Australian data she shows that business corporations, through mergers, are now responsible for providing both CAM and orthodox therapies in private hospitals, and several corporations are producing both healthcare products and standard pharmaceuticals. CAM has thus followed orthodox medicine and moved from a cottage industry to a mature market sector.

In the third and final part, 'Boundary Contestation in the Workplace', we turn our attention to the plurality of experts who bring therapeutic options into the medical marketplace to be assessed, controlled and ultimately to be consumed. Increasingly, the nature of the CAM provider has become ever more diverse, difficult to stereotype and characterised by a location at the intersection of professional and cultural worlds. Despite this, the section opens with an argument by Coulter (Chapter 6) that clear epistemological differences between the 'sectors' remain, and that it is these that explain, or at least contribute to, the problems with integration that continue to be found in practice. He presents an argument that systems theory offers a potential means through which persistent conflicts can be resolved.

Having opened the section with this overarching discussion of the philosophical underpinnings of orthodox and non-orthodox provision, the book is rounded off with three chapters, each of which looks at a specific group of providers: Chapter 7, CAM practitioners (Boon et al.); Chapter 8, GPs who use CAM (Adams); and, Chapter 9, CAM nurses (Adams and Tovey). While these groups of providers may, superficially, be seen to be in one camp or another, these chapters highlight the way in which boundaries and identities appear to be increasingly blurred.

Boon and her colleagues draw on empirical work in Canada, studying naturopaths, homeopaths and traditional Chinese medical practitioners to illustrate the complexity of the relationship between the state and professionalising processes. They show that each group sought statutory self-regulation from the state to achieve occupational closure. However, to achieve this they needed to demonstrate unity among their practitioners and for some therapies this has proved very difficult. Further, even if unity was achieved, there had to be a clear niche in the healthcare system into which they could fit as a specialist provider for them to be successful.

But, of course, therapies are no longer the preserve of 'CAM practitioners' alone. Across advanced societies, practitioners trained in, and frequently still practising, orthodox approaches are selectively embracing or appropriating techniques to form a part of their therapeutic options. Because of their role as the first point of contact, and because of their retention of status as 'head' of the primary care team, GPs who practise CAM are clearly worthy of attention. In recent years we have seen a smattering of studies looking at this group of practitioners. In this area, as with others, we are far from achieving a uniform interpretation of events. In Chapter 8, Adams illustrates how GP therapists demarcate their identity and practice from that of non-medically qualified therapists situated in the private health care sector. He suggests, from his exploratory study of GPs in Scotland, that such boundary-work, delineating complementary and alternative therapy, helps these doctors claim an essential role in the provision of good, effective CAM practice.

Although GPs may have attracted much of the research attention, it is actually another orthodox healthcare profession – nursing – that would appear to be, both numerically and ideologically, most at one with CAM. However, as Adams and Tovey discuss in Chapter 9, this enthusiasm has, to date, largely avoided critical sociological commentary, with published work on CAM nursing thus far largely remaining the province of 'insiders'. The argument made in this chapter is that, in order to begin to unravel this apparent affinity, there is a need to shift from a supportive advocacy to a critical engagement that challenges many taken-for-granted assumptions about the CAM/nursing relationship and interface. A framework whereby this may be advanced is outlined.

To summarise, at the time of writing, the under-researched nature of CAM is becoming increasingly widely recognised, and strategies are emerging from policy-makers as a first step to addressing this (Department of Health 2002). However, in the pursuit of 'answers' to policy questions (Does it work? Is it safe? How can be it integrated?), there is a danger that research questions become ever more narrowly conceptualised and the means through which answers are sought (for example the randomised controlled trial) become ever more tightly prescribed. This book has been produced with a view to addressing crucial issues (some seemingly familiar from the policy agenda and some not) from a broader, less immediately utilitarian approach: one influenced by the pursuit of critical, sociologically informed understanding.

Notes

1 Complementary and alternative medicine refers to those healing practices and medications that are not part of orthodox medicine. As will become clear in this book, what constitutes such practices and medications is both temporally and spatially variable. It is also the subject of considerable contestation. However, the term and its acronym CAM are now the accepted terminology in academic writing on the topic; consequently, we use them in this book.
2 By advanced societies, we refer to those societies that have strong tertiary economic sectors and, importantly for our purposes, a medical system that is dominated by orthodox medicine (sometimes called Western medicine or bio-medicine). The countries in that category examined in this book are the English-speaking countries of Australia, Canada, New Zealand, the UK and the USA. There are many interesting issues to do with the relationship between Western medicine, traditional medicines and 'international CAMs' in poorer countries, but they are not addressed here.

References

Department of Health (2002) *Developing Research Capacity for Complementary and Alternative Medicine: A strategy for action*, Leeds: Department of Health.

Downey, P. (1997) *Homeopathy for the Primary Care Team: A guide for GPs, midwives, district nurses and other health professionals*, Oxford: Butterworth Heinemann.

Easthope, G., Tranter, B. and Gill, G. (1998) 'Acupuncture in Australian general practice: practitioner characteristics', *Medical Journal of Australia* 169,4: 197–2000.

Ernst, E., Pittler, M.H., Stevinson, X., White, A.R. and Eisenberg, D. (2001) *The Desktop Guide to CAM*, Edinburgh: Mosby.

House of Lords (2000) *Complementary and Alternative Medicine*, London: House of Lords.

Schepers, R.M.J. and Hermans, H.E.G.M. (1999) 'The medical profession and alternative medicine in the Netherlands: its history and recent development', *Social Science and Medicine* 48,3: 343–52.

Tanvir, J. (2001) *Complementary Medicine: A practical guide*, Oxford: Butterworth Heinemann.

Tovey, P. and Adams, J. (2001) 'Primary care as intersecting social worlds', *Social Science and Medicine* 52: 695–706.

Trevelyan, J. and Booth, B. (1994) *Complementary Medicine for Nurses, Midwives and Health Visitors*, London: Macmillan.

Vickers, A. (1993) *Massage and Aromatherapy: A guide for health professionals*, London: Chapman and Hall.

Ullman, D. (1993) 'The mainstreaming of alternative medicine', *Healthcare Forum Journal*. Nov/Dec: 24–30.

Wardwell, W. (1994) 'Alternative medicine in the United States', *Social Science and Medicine* 38,8: 1061–8.

Willis, E. (1989) *Medical Dominance*, rev. edn, Sydney: Allen & Unwin.

Part I

Consumption in cultural context

Chapter 1

Consumption as activism

An examination of CAM as part of the consumer movement in health

Melinda Goldner

Is CAM a social movement?

CAM is more often defined as a set of diverse techniques or beliefs than as a social movement: techniques and beliefs that vary widely in their use and acceptability. However, Alster believes CAM does constitute a movement, because there are:

> common beliefs about health and some common goals regarding health-care. Furthermore, the existence of holistic journals and organisations indicates that the theme provides a common ground for diverse groups. . . . 'Movement' probably comes as close as any available term to describing the collective activity of the holists.
>
> (Alster 1989: 47)

He goes on to argue that the CAM movement has coalesced around slogans, such as 'you are responsible for your own health', 'health is more than the absence of disease', and 'a good practitioner must care for the whole person' (Alster 1989: 54–5). Such beliefs and slogans provide a common sense of collective identity. Goldstein suggests that these values and beliefs allow people within such a diverse movement to 'find a common sense of identity' (Goldstein 1999: 136). This identity allows diverse people to identify with a seemingly cohesive movement, even when they may never interact or never agree entirely on such elements as goals. It is this collective identity, not social movement organisations, which provides cohesion for the movement.

The CAM movement, it is suggested, operates on two levels simultaneously (Schneirov and Geczik 1996). First, it acts as an interest group through lobby groups such as the Nutrition Health Alliance and professional associations such as the American Holistic Medical Association (Goldstein *et al.* 1987; Wolpe 1990). Interest groups try to mobilise support through advocating legislative reform, educating the general public, acquiring resources and developing coalitions. Second, the movement operates in submerged networks of social movement communities (Buechler 1990) where activists attempt to create and sustain an alternative way of life, especially through sharing information. This information is frequently mundane, such as what foods a healthy person should eat. However, '[it is] often placed within the broader context of a moral crusade for a deeper and more fundamental change in basic values and assumptions' (Goldstein 1999: 136). The various submerged networks have played a larger role within the CAM movement than the interest groups just described above.

Though some activists still advocate CAM as an alternative to Western medicine (Goldner 2001), the CAM movement has been increasingly successful with the goal of integration into Western medicine so that 'the question for healthcare systems has become not *if*, but *when* they will get involved' (emphasis added) (Larson 2001: 6). In response to the increased numbers of consumers who are using CAM, the number of community hospitals in the USA offering CAM increased by 25 per cent from 1998 to 1999 (American Hospital Association's Survey of Hospitals as cited in Larson 2001: 6). Medi-Cal, which is California's version of Medicaid, now allows acupuncturists to serve as primary practitioners for enrollees (Baer *et al.* 1998a, 1998b). Any facility that receives accreditation from the Joint Commission on Accreditation of Healthcare Organizations (JCAHO) must educate patients about pain management with CAM. Referring to this policy, Weeks says 'this is no longer just a consumer movement . . . the police power in the industry is now involved . . . [but] you need ongoing marketing pressure [to sustain these practices financially]' (as quoted in Larson 2001: 9).

These various writings suggest that CAM consumers may be part of a social movement. To ascertain whether such consumers do or do not constitute a movement, I conducted an exploratory study of CAM consumers. The study is detailed below.

The study

The study was based on interviews with individuals in two locations. The first sample consisted of consumers from the San Francisco, California Bay area. This area was chosen as it has been argued that the CAM movement in the USA originated and flourished there (Baer *et al.* 1998a, 1998b). In order to show activism in other locations, the second sample consists of consumers from the Capital District around Albany, New York. I rely upon data from consumers; however, I also include some information on how practitioners are active as consumers.

The Bay area sample comes from a larger study of forty people: thirty practitioners and ten clients. Though I highlight the ways in which some of the thirty practitioners are active in the CAM movement as consumers, I mainly rely upon interviews with ten clients; two of whom were in the process of training to become alternative practitioners. Since I only wanted to interview people who used CAM, I located all forty respondents through posting fliers in alternative clinics and other public locations, asking clinics for recommendations from their client lists, and then using snowball sampling. Respondents were more likely to have used acupuncture, chiropractic and herbs. On average, consumers had used seven modalities; however, there was one individual who used over thirty techniques. Since I include some data on practitioners, the following are the demographic characteristics of all forty people interviewed. Respondents were overwhelmingly female (73 per cent) and Caucasian (97 per cent), and ranged in age from 35 to 63 (mean age = 47). All respondents had taken some college courses, and twenty-eight (70 per cent) finished some graduate work or earned graduate degrees. Religious or spiritual affiliation varied greatly, though ten (26 per cent) said they had no affiliation with any religion. Sixteen (40 per cent) of the respondents were currently married, though an additional thirteen (33 per cent) were previously married. Finally, respondents did not report their incomes accurately enough to ascertain a reliable range or mean.

The Capital District sample consisted of nine consumers. Three were also alternative practitioners; however, I highlight the ways in which they are active as consumers. These respondents were also located by posting fliers in clinics and utilising snowball sampling. There were four men and five women with an average age of 45 (range from 27 to 57). All were non-Hispanic white, except for one who identified as Hispanic. Four were married, three were never married and one was widowed. Three respondents had children. All respondents had some exposure to college courses, and all but one had a college degree. One also had a graduate degree. One was unemployed, while the rest were employed in a variety of jobs. Three did not identify with any religion, one identified as Pagan, another Jewish, and two as Wiccan. On average, respondents regularly used 3.2 forms of CAM with herbs, chiropractic, acupuncture and Reiki as the most popular.

Results

Most respondents identified themselves as activists within a larger CAM movement. Their activism started from their use of these techniques. They began to experience results and identify with the beliefs behind these techniques. Their activism then extended to educating others about CAM. No one in this study used CAM exclusively; rather, they desired integration with Western medicine. Consequently, they engaged in tactics that attempted to change institutions, not just individuals. For example, they requested insurance reimbursement and asked physicians, and their respective healthcare organisations, to be more accepting of CAM.

Shared actions and beliefs

In the Bay area sample, most believed there is a CAM movement, and two-thirds of the consumers identified as activists. All of the respondents in the Capital District sample believed there is a CAM movement and all identified as activists. Thus the majority of consumers in both samples believed there is a CAM movement, and most identified as activists within it. However, one Capital District respondent qualified her answer by saying, 'I wouldn't [consider myself an activist], because I think activists are more vocal . . . writing letters, lobbying . . . [however] within my own healthcare I would consider myself one, but I keep it to myself more'. Such a response is indicative of the different strategies and tactics that are used in this movement in comparison to most social movements. In particular, activism in the CAM movement often involves individual acts such as using these techniques, educating others and seeking insurance reimbursement. Many respondents noted how different these tactics are in comparison to other social movements that are more likely to utilise collective activities, such as public protests.

Most respondents believed that using CAM and improving their own health are forms of activism. One male said '[I] consider myself active [in the movement], since I use a lot of these services'. He believed that consumers can have 'a big impact, because you've got more people using [CAM]'. Another respondent, who is a practitioner, stated:

> it starts within each of us. It has to begin internally, I think, but then if we can help one another and influence the culture and the world we are in, then that's fantastic. That's what I hope for too.

A male consumer expanded on this idea:

> I know for me I definitely want to use [CAM] as a tool for empowerment and politics . . . [In] health movements, you work on yourself first, and then work on other people . . . I feel really strongly about that – that you need to work on yourself whether it [is] mental, physical, or spiritual issues, and whether [you use] Qigong or another form of medicine. Whatever will help you strive to be the best you can be so you can be more effective in your daily life and help really make the change.

Consumers are often profoundly affected by CAM, not just because of the results, but because they agree with the beliefs behind these techniques. Core beliefs include defining health holistically as well-being rather than the absence of disease, stressing individual responsibility for health, and using 'natural' therapeutic techniques (Kopelman and Moskop 1981).

These beliefs provide coherence for the movement, because they allow activists to recognise a shared ideology.

In terms of holism, some respondents simply stressed that CAM looks at the 'whole' person, not just one part of that person. In dealing with health and illness, this means that mental, emotional and spiritual concerns are just as important as physical symptoms and disease. Other respondents referred to specific aspects that CAM addresses, such as one woman who said that people's feelings impact their health. The goal of health then is well-being, not simply the absence of disease. Many used the term 'balance' to describe what they meant by well-being. They strive for balance in their lives even when disease is not present. Others explained well-being by distinguishing between healing and curing. Even when people have a disease that cannot be cured, they can improve their lives spiritually, emotionally, mentally and socially. They experience healing. The focus on holism and well-being requires a different relationship between the practitioner and patient.

A patient's relationship with the practitioner is different because of CAM's expectation that consumers will take individual responsibility for their health, thus become empowered. (For a detailed elaboration of the concept of responsibility see Hughes, Chapter 2.) Individual responsibility means different things to different people. In the extreme it can mean that 'if you accept responsibility for your health, you have to also accept responsibility for having allowed the disease, creating the disease, or gotten the disease, and that can be something people don't want to do'. Others simply take this to mean that they need to take responsibility for finding the solution, rather than for having created the problem. Many consumers felt empowered by this. One informant even mentioned that he uses CAM as a 'tool for empowerment'. Several respondents mentioned that being empowered to take responsibility could mean that, rather than simply taking a pill given to them by a physician, they might need to change their lifestyle.

Consumers in this study believed that CAM utilises more natural treatments, prevention and lifestyle changes. Comparing what they perceive as the more 'natural' treatments in CAM to Western medicine, one male said 'you almost can't trust regular doctors because you don't want to be drugged up all your life'. Since many agreed that 'a lot of times most of my ailments are ultimately lifestyle or stress-related', possible treatments included changing jobs, seeking counselling or reducing stress. Given this belief, another woman stated 'sometimes healing isn't about taking a pill. Sometimes you just need to go get mad at someone, instead of holding it in. Illness will grow and grow if you don't let that go'. Another said:

> Instead of taking a Valium, come in and talk about your feelings. Come and get some support. People are beginning to realise that your emo-

tions, instead of being dulled, need to be expressed if people are going to survive with any degree of health at the end of it.

As these quotes suggest, many consumers interviewed stressed that CAM can help to get at the 'root of the problem' or prevent disease entirely.

Educating others

As many respondents said, people see results, and then want to share these techniques and beliefs with others; their activism extends beyond personal consumption. Respondents emphasised that CAM is not a typical social movement, given its grassroots nature. One noted that there are pockets of users, especially in places like New York City, San Francisco and Boston, but she could not think of anyone who acts as a lead spokesperson for the national movement. Others could not think of any national organisations that are part of the movement. With no identifiable place to turn to, one activist noted that you have to talk to people to find information on CAM.

This is why one of the most critical tactics of the movement is what activists call 'word of mouth'. Many mentioned that a family member or friend's recommendation was the reason they first tried CAM. Now they encourage others to use these techniques. One woman said that 'for the most part' patients tell their family members and 'bring them into consciousness of it. . . . Word of mouth is very important [because it leads to openness to try these techniques]'. Another respondent added that she considered herself an activist to the extent that she tries to 'encourage others to look at alternatives'.

Respondents reported that many people have heard of CAM, but do not use it until someone personally recommends it. As one respondent explained, 'most of the people that I've spoken to are a little bit leery about alternative medicine. Once I tell them that it's very effective, then they catch on'. Another pointed out that someone can read an article about CAM, but they will not try it until a friend recommends it. She went on to say that her friend changed her mind. Since her consumption has 'had a positive influence [since she says she is healthier now than she was twenty years ago], I would hope that [I could do that for others]'. One woman said that of 'the people I've gotten on my side who were non-believers, I wasn't able to get them on my side until they actually tried these techniques for themselves'. She clarified that consumption not only lays the groundwork for belief in CAM, but that you need consumption to be an activist. Even activism of practitioners, she says, stems from their role as consumers, not practitioners.

Many respondents noted that word of mouth is currently the most effective strategy to get people to use CAM. First, you can rely on the trust and respect within that personal relationship. One woman stated 'because of the friendship with this person, I have the opportunity to educate her. The way I think of it is that she'll go, "You know I was talking to some-body". . . . Then that's just word of mouth.' Second, respondents believe that they are likely to see results and become believers. One man said, 'so a lot of it depends upon [CAM] being available, and being not only socially acceptable, but people seeing that it makes a difference'. Third, some respondents believe that word of mouth is more effective than the internet or other forms of media, because they believe that public information is often false or misleading. As one respondent explained:

> [People] don't feel knowledgeable enough about these techniques, so they have to rely on someone. It's worse than getting their car fixed [in terms of how little they know]. So the public does have to be educated. But where do they get their information? Listening to the TV, they won't get the story due to who does the advertising.

Though some of this information is accurate, the varying reliability of information has led activists to pursue other strategies beyond using and advocating CAM.

Changing healthcare institutions

When asked whether activists were interested in changing individuals or institutions, one woman said 'a little bit of both'. Another argued that you can not rely on the government to advocate CAM, so you need a strong grassroots component to achieve institutional change. Part of the structural changes activists seek is insurance reimbursement. One respondent talked about this in detail, because he worked for an insurance company. He saw lots of subscribers send in requests for reimbursement for their use of CAM. A couple of respondents said that it is more difficult to change insur-ance practices since the movement operates on the grassroots level, and not through more formal social movement organisations. Yet, as one respon-dent said, 'once the HMOs [Health Maintenance Organisations] see that these alternative treatments can actually help people, then they are going to be more susceptible to want to accept them'.

Some activists turn their consumption of CAM into a more critical stance towards Western medicine. One respondent believed that:

> There is pressure from patients. Society is unhappy. They don't want to just get sick. The baby boomers aren't accepting the inevitability of their bodies falling apart at fifty as earlier generations did. And they won't just rely on their doctors. So a large population of people are saying they aren't happy, questioning doctors, and wanting to stay well.

When asked about the impact of his consumption, one said:

> I would say it would have a big impact since it would tend to lean me away [from] the factory system of regular doctors. . . . In fact, I just changed my primary care physician because I was not happy at all with the service I was getting from the family practice department over at [a local hospital], because they made you feel impersonal.

Another woman said that the only way in which she sees CAM as a social movement is that people are now insisting they get 'service and value for their dollars'.

Although many respondents complained about orthodox medicine, they did not reject it. In fact, all of the respondents used Western medicine, especially when facing emergencies or acute problems. Most respondents believed that the goal of the movement is to incorporate CAM into Western medicine. When one respondent was asked where the movement was heading, she said, 'I think that we're going to move toward the idea of complementary medicine . . . the kinds of clinics that would mix MDs with other licensed caregivers'. Given their desire for integration, one said that her activism includes the fact that she is willing to talk about these techniques with physicians. In her words, she 'acts as a consumer'. She went on to say that 'we are a more consumer-oriented society', so doctors have to 'prove their worth' to her. This means they must 'learn a little bit more [about CAM, and] accept a little bit more'.

Respondents credited consumers for some of the changes taking place within Western medicine. In addition to obtaining insurance reimbursement, respondents found that some physicians and nurses were recommending and even practising CAM. Many noted that these changes have taken years to develop. One said, 'it took years to realise there is an alternative to Western medicine, [but] now it's big business'. Another stated that, 'I saw some statistic published recently about people spending more of their discretionary dollars on alternative care than on Western care. Doctors want a piece of that market. It's a highly motivating factor'. Respondents were clear on the role of consumers. One said, 'the public is the driver', and another said, 'it's the public that are driving the changes' within Western medicine.

Conclusion

Consumers have played a major role within the CAM movement. They have been an integral part of this grassroots movement, given the scarcity of national leaders and formal social movement organisations that could take the lead, as well as in the predominantly market-based healthcare system in the USA. Activists are using various forms of CAM, telling their friends to use CAM, asking their physicians to be open to these techniques, and demanding insurance reimbursement. Though these are individual acts, consumers believe they are participating in a form of activism. They feel connected to a larger movement, given their shared ideology, tactics and goals. Consumers are having a collective impact that is political, not just medical.

There are some possible problems that could result from the movement's emphasis on consumerism. In particular, the movement could suffer from a commercialisation that leads to inappropriate usage, co-optation and problems of equity in access. Yet, the CAM movement is creating significant and rapid changes within the American healthcare system.

The CAM movement is a fluid movement (Gusfield 1994). Though fluid movements are based on everyday actions of individuals, activists believe that each action is 'taken with the recognition that it is not isolated and individualistic' (Gusfield 1994: 66). Being an activist within a fluid movement reflects a commitment to the movement's ideas. As noted earlier, slogans such as 'you are responsible for your own health' and 'health is more than the absence of disease' are popular and are widely repeated 'both inside the movement and beyond its confines as well' (Alster 1989: 54). Most importantly, they provide cohesion for activists who are often engaging in individual forms of activism, and allow the amorphous movement to speak with a more unified voice.

CAM is a movement without recognised national leaders or a formal social movement organisation. Two points can be made here. First,

> in terms of leadership, the holistic health network, heavily influenced by the anti-bureaucratic ethos of 1960s radicalism, emphasises democratic participation as well as group solidarity. The leadership is quite self-effacing and wary of taking on too much responsibility.
> (Evans as paraphrased in Schneirov and Geczik 1996: 635)

Even advocates of integrative medicine, such as Andrew Weil, Deepak Chopra, Herbert Benson, Alice Domar, Dean Ornish, Mehmet Oz and Rachel Naomi Remen do not typically identify as activists within the CAM movement. More importantly, very few respondents in this study mentioned these individuals, and the majority could not name any national leaders. Second, although formal social movement organisations or interest groups do exist that advocate legislative reform, educate the general public, acquire resources, and develop coalitions (some examples include the Nutrition Health Alliance and Citizens for Health, as well as professional associations such as the American Holistic Medical Association (Goldstein *et al.* 1987; Wolpe 1990) the majority of respondents did not mention these national organisations.

The centrality of consumers in the CAM movement in the USA is because of the primarily market-based healthcare system there. Markets rely on the numerous independent decisions and acts of producers and consumers. This system allows entrepreneurs to market their products directly to consumers. For example, when the American Congress passed the Dietary Supplement Health and Education Act (DSHEA) in 1994, manufacturers were allowed to market a variety of herbs, supplements and vitamins without obtaining approval from the Food and Drug Administration. They were allowed to claim beneficial effects as long as they did not claim to treat a specific disease.

> Largely as a result of this new freedom of manufacturers and distributors to make sweeping but purposely vague claims, the average American is now exposed to a steady diet of advertising for all manner of supplements (especially herbal preparations), which in turn has led to a dramatic increase in their consumption.
>
> (Reisser *et al.* 2001: 13)

Producers clearly have the ability to persuade consumers to try their products. However, market-based systems also allow consumers to purchase or reject specific goods and services. Consumption of CAM in the USA has increased dramatically through a series of independent decisions made by consumers, as well as word of mouth. One male respondent likened it to 'rabbits breeding in a cage', since the information can multiply quickly. In order to maintain financial solvency, any producer has to follow these consumption decisions closely. In the USA, this means that many healthcare organisations, from hospitals to insurance companies, pay attention to the increased consumption of CAM. Though primarily a decentralised system, the US government has stepped in where necessary to regulate CAM, since there is this large-scale consumption.

Western medicine in the USA has responded to the CAM movement, given the power of consumers. In particular, physicians and hospital staff have listened to the majority of activists who desire CAM's integration into Western medicine. Already:

> Forty-two states require private insurers to cover chiropractic treatments, and two states (Washington and Wisconsin) require insurers to offer coverage at an extra charge; six states mandate acupuncture coverage . . . two states require massage coverage, and four naturopathy. . . . Medicare covers chiropractic treatment under certain circumstances. And now employers – under pressure to please workers in today's tight labour market – are including CAM in the plans they offer their employees. From 1990 to 1997 the percentage of employer-provided health plans that covered some alternative therapies

rose from 30 per cent to 70 per cent. Two-thirds of HMOs now offer CAM.

(Lee and Ryan 2000: 179)

As Reisser *et al.* (2001: 20) argue, insurance companies are increasingly covering these techniques, in large part, because 'the customers want it'. Of course, physicians maintain a great deal of control. For example, many insurance companies will only cover complementary techniques if referred or provided by a physician (Lee and Ryan 2000). Yet, consumers are having a collective impact. Dr Andrew Weil argues that:

It is still a consumer-led movement, but it's gaining a real response from academic medicine. At this point, I think it's unstoppable and that it will result in a transformed system, including the system of medical education. Much needs to happen before that comes to pass, but I clearly see us moving in that direction.

(As quoted in Horrigan 2001)

Consumers may have fuelled the growing acceptance of CAM, yet their dramatic consumption patterns may lead to commercialisation that could have negative consequences for the movement. First, anyone marketing these techniques could exaggerate results in order to attract consumers. Reissman provides the example of vitamin B-12, which has been marketed as being a way to increase energy. He says this 'is based essentially on the fact that it has this effect on highly anemic individuals – an example of extrapolating from the extremes to the masses' (Reissman 1994: 55). It would be detrimental to the movement if consumers begin to use these techniques inappropriately, because this could lead to a lack of results and frustration. Second, there is the possibility that these techniques could become co-opted as they enter the mainstream (Goldner 2000). More physicians are seeking training in CAM. An estimated 3,000 American physicians integrate acupuncture into their practices (Langone 1996: 40), and an estimated one-third of homeopaths are physicians or osteopaths (Dranov 1996: 96). If these physicians do not use these techniques in accordance with the beliefs outlined above, some respondents believe they 'won't get results'. If this proves true, then this could frustrate consumers and do more harm than good for the movement. Co-optation occurs in other forms. Goldstein (1999) uses the example of chiropractic work to illustrate how a modality can be restricted when insurance companies begin to reimburse the technique, because they limit the type of conditions it can treat and number of visits. Some activists would argue that these restrictions prevent consumers from experiencing the full range of benefits possible. If research bears this out, then the movement could be negatively affected.

There is also the possibility that issues of equity and access worsen as commercialisation intensifies. Since insurance coverage is still partial, most consumers have to pay out-of-pocket for these techniques. This has largely restricted their use to the upper and middle class. Since CAM is 'not really open to the general public', part of one consumer's activism is to make it more available. Third-party payment is the most viable option. Until this happens, basic laws of supply and demand dictate that the price demanded for these techniques will be out of reach for many consumers, especially as the commercialisation of these techniques increases their popularity.

> What is unique is that a consumer movement like CAM is assisted by consumers who fall outside the movement. Though the majority of respondents in this study identified explicitly as activists within the CAM movement, many people use CAM without identifying in this way. In fluid movements, 'membership is also fluid. Movements can have consequences and influence behavior without the kind of commitment or ideological agreement that is often posited for them.
>
> (Gusfield 1994: 64)

Some individuals may never identify as activists within the CAM movement, nor even agree with the ideology behind the techniques, yet their consumption is still influential. Consumer movements have the best of both worlds.

This chapter has been based on the results from a small-scale, essentially exploratory study. Future research needs to find out more about the large group of consumers who are using CAM without adopting its beliefs. We need to find out how many consumers identify as activists within the CAM movement, and whether or not it will continue to matter whether or not they do so. We need to ascertain how many consumers agree with the ideas behind the techniques. The full impact of consumers, both individually and collectively, needs to be assessed in the predominantly market-based system of the USA. Finally, studies should also examine whether most consumer movements are decentralised, fluid and amorphous.

References and select bibliography

Alster, K.B. (1989) *The Holistic Health Movement*, Tuscaloosa: The University of Alabama Press.

Atlanta Constitution, The (2000) 'Close to home where you live: your voice, your questions, your community news', October 17, C2.

Baer, H.A., Hays, J., McClendon, N., McGoldrick, N. and Vespucci, R. (1998a) 'The holistic health movement in the San Francisco Bay Area: some preliminary observations', *Social Science & Medicine* 47: 1495–501.

Baer, H.A., Jen, C., Tanassi, L.M., Tsia, C. and Wahbeh, H. (1998b) 'The drive for professionalisation in acupuncture: a preliminary view from the San Francisco Bay Area', *Social Science & Medicine* 46: 533–7.

Bennett, J. and Brown, C.M. (2000) 'Use of herbal remedies by patients in a health maintenance organization', *Journal of the American Pharmaceutical Association* 40: 353–8.

Buechler, S. (1990) *Women's Movements in the United states*, New Brunswick, NJ: Rutgers University Press.

Dranov, P. (1996) 'Alternative medicine: what helps, what hurts', *Ladies Home Journal* November: 94–9.

Goldner, M. (2000) 'Integrative medicine: issues to consider in this emerging form of health care', *Research in the Sociology of Health Care* 17: 213–33.

Goldner, M. (2001) 'Expanding political opportunities and changing collective identities in the complementary and alternative medicine movement', *Political Opportunities, Social Movements, and Democratization* 23: 69–102.

Goldstein, M.S. (1999) *Alternative Health Care: medicine, miracle, or mirage*, Philadelphia: Temple University Press.

Goldstein, M.S. (2000) 'The growing acceptance of complementary and alternative medicine', in Bird, C.E. , Conrad, P. and Fremont, A.M. (eds) *Handbook of Medical Sociology*, Upper Saddle River, NJ: Prentice Hall.

Goldstein, M.S., Jaffe, D.T., Sutherland, C. and Wilson, J. (1987) 'Holistic physicians: implications for the study of the medical profession', *Journal of Health and Social Behavior* 28: 103–19.

Gulla, J., Singer, A.J. and Gaspari, R. (2001) 'Herbal use in ED patients', *SAEM 2001 Annual Meeting Abstracts* 8: 450.

Gusfield, J.R. (1994) 'The reflexivity of social movements: collective behavior and mass society theory revisited', in Larana, E., Johnston, H. and Gusfield, J.R. (eds) *New Social Movements: from ideology to identity*, Philadelphia: Temple University Press.

Horrigan, B. (2000) 'National integrative medicine organisation formed', *Alternative Therapies in Health and Medicine* 6: 30.

Horrigan, B. (2001) 'Andrew Weil, on integrative medicine and the nature of reality', *Alternative Therapies in Health and Medicine* 7: 96–104.

Kelner, M. and Wellman, B. (1997) 'Health care and consumer choice: medical and alternative therapies', *Social Science & Medicine* 45: 203–12.

Kopelman, L. and Moskop, J. (1981) 'The holistic health movement: a survey and critique', *The Journal of Medicine and Philosophy* 6: 209–35.

Langone, J. (1996) 'Challenging the mainstream', *TIME*, Special Issue, Fall: 40–3.

Larson, L. (2001) 'Natural selection', *Trustee* 54: 6–12.

Lee, J. and Ryan, B. (2000) 'Easing the pain', *Money* 29: 179–80.

Reisser, P.C., Mabe, D. and Velarde, R. (2001) *Examining Alternative Medicine: an Inside Look at the Benefits & Risks*, Downers Grove, Illinois: InterVarsity Press.

Reissman, F. (1994) 'Alternative health movements', *Social Policy* 24: 53–7.

Schneirov, M. and Geczik, J.D. (1996) 'A diagnosis for our times: alternative health's submerged networks and the transformation of identities', *The Sociological Quarterly* 37: 627–44.

Shelton, D.L. (2000) 'The herbal hype of dietary supplements', *American Medical News* 43: 27–8.

Taylor, V. and Whittier, N. (1992) 'Collective identity in social movement communities', in Morris, A. and Mueller, C.M. (eds) *Frontiers in Social Movement Theory*, New Haven: Yale University Press.

Weldon, M. (2000) 'A spiritual way to look at medicine', *Chicago Tribune* July 5, 8.3.

Wolpe, P. (1990) 'The holistic heresy: strategies of ideological challenge', *Social Science & Medicine* 31: 913–23.

Chapter 2

Health as individual responsibility

Possibilities and personal struggle

Kahryn Hughes

Introduction: the body-as-project – bodies, health and identity

Following related discussion earlier in this Part, this chapter presents a sociological consideration of the ways in which people consulting CAM practitioners are encouraged to exercise individual responsibility in the process of their healthcare.[1] It has been argued that, underpinning philosophies of the New Age culture, is the assumption that every human individual is essentially capable of perfect health and mental adjustment if only s/he is prepared to take responsibility for her/his own health. Such a philosophy, it is held, is responsible for the increasing trend in people paying privately for CAMs (Coward 1989: 11). People's expectations, it is argued, about their role in their health and healthcare have changed, and this role is something CAMs are predicated on: namely, a proactive, empowered and responsible 'client' role. Therefore, exploring this trend in increasing acceptance of and drive towards self-responsibility is, in part, an exploration of broader societal trends. In particular, this philosophical development has been linked to 'being committed to our bodies' (Coward 1989), underpinned by discourses of the 'civilised body' (Elias 1978) which conceive of 'the body-as-project' (Shilling 1993). Susceptible to illness and disease, 'the body' is subjected to regulatory regimes involving diet and exercise (Shilling 1993; Bordo 1995) in order to prevent, or reduce the risk of, illness and to subvert the possible pathologies to which we are predisposed (Martin 1987; Ehrenreich and English 1988; Bordo 1995). Perceiving 'risks' to our health through smoking, eating (too much, not the right food), exercise (not doing any, doing too much, going too far), and seeking out healthcare is a route for self-determination (I am this rather than that) and is part of engaging in a set of practices in the ongoing constitution of one's identity (this is who I am) (see Foucault 1990). In other words, seeking healthcare and being involved in healthcare significantly contributes to the processes of identity constitution in which we are engaged.

Historically, much literature on CAMs and biomedicine has focused on differentiating between their different philosophies of health, healing, healthcare and identity (see Coulter, Chapter 6). In this chapter, analysing the discourses constituting the patient's role and responsibility in their healthcare, I will explore the ways in which CAMs and biomedicine can be seen to be increasingly converging (helping working towards overcoming the simplified distinction between CAMs and orthodox medicine). In particular, I will discuss the ways in which the patient's role is constituted across a range of CAMs and will later contextualise this discussion with some analyses of the central discourses of patients' and carers' roles in the UK National Health Service (NHS), which is currently undergoing a process of 'modernisation'. This later part of the chapter will concentrate on the processes whereby the individual's identity and corresponding 'normative rights' for their healthcare (Sevenhuijsen 2000) involves increased 'empowerment' and 'autonomy' in biomedical philosophies of healthcare. Further, analyses will focus on discourses of patient identity, responsibilities, rights and healthcare participation in state discourses of health, referring specifically to the NHS Plan, the Patient's Charter and the proposed NHS Charter as some of the most recent (2002) examples. Here, I will also consider the usefulness of conceiving of patient/user engagement in public and private care settings as a form of citizenship activity (Sevenhuijsen 2000).

Empirical studies

The following discussion is based on empirical research undertaken in a Local Health Authority in West Yorkshire, where the aim was to explore the notion of 'holism' in CAMs (Hughes *et al.* 1997; Long *et al.* 2000) and on research in London with clients with HIV/AIDS who used CAM practitioners, exploring with them reasons for consulting CAM practitioners and their experiences of CAM. Both studies employed in-depth interviews and focus groups with patients and CAM practitioners, both in the NHS and in private practice. In the West Yorkshire study we used a grounded theory approach, involving in-depth interviews with patients who had been referred by their GPs to CAM practitioners, with whom the GPs had already developed a commissioning model whereby they could purchase packages of CAM for patients with common mental health problems. In-depth interviews were also undertaken with the GPs, the CAM practitioners, non-referred patients of these practitioners with similar conditions and practitioners of CAMs within the NHS, such as GPs using acupuncture and nurses using reflexology and aromatherapy. Focus groups with both the CAM practitioners and NHS practitioners of CAMs were also held to check back on analyses of the interview data. The study in London was solely focus group work with a series of groups of gay men with HIV/AIDS, women with HIV/AIDS and the broad range of complementary practitioners working with these groups (four groups in total). In both studies, in either interview or focus group, we explored the patient's role and responsibility, which emerged as central to the participants' experiences, understandings and philosophies of CAM. Subsequent analyses of the data from these studies have varied according to purpose. For the reports to the commissioning health authority, we undertook content analysis. In this chapter, however, discourse analysis (Banister *et al.* 1995) has also been used.

Theory as method, method as theory

'Discourse', drawing on the work of Foucault (1972), is capable of constituting the subjects of which it speaks; it organises and informs power/knowledge networks, and creates the conditions for localised power relations. This chapter develops Foucault's work on the care of the self (Foucault 1990), by exploring the ways in which identities are constituted and maintained through particular organisational discourses and practices. Using Foucault, discourse analysis is both a process of theory production and a method of inquiry. This approach enables us to engage with empirical research on 'local levels', such as therapeutic encounters with CAM practitioners, and more precisely at the level of 'events' or *practices* (see also Fisher and Groce 1985; Nettleton 1991). Consequently, by exploring the ways in which the patient is encouraged to engage in and take responsibility for their health and healthcare, and the philosophies underpinning CAM and the organisational features or practices of CAM based on or contradictory to these philosophies, I seek to develop an understanding of the type of patient constituted within CAMs. In particular, by examining the discourses employed in the interviews and focus groups emerging from these studies, I explore the ways in which individual responsibility is constituted in the context of the individual's state of health, their recovery and their (non) engagement in CAM healthcare settings. The following discussion will explore the different responsibilities accruing at each stage of the patient's process through treatment: becoming ill, seeking and/or participating in treatment, what the treatment does, recovery, success and ending the treatment.

Becoming ill: who is becoming ill and what is responsible?

Analysis of contemporary health promotion discourse in the UK NHS reveals a tension in the ascription of agency and responsibility for ill health (Connolly and Emmel forthcoming). Specifically, tensions emerge between approaches of 'expert/evidence' models of public health, where the focus is on individuals and populations and public health action which includes prescribing personal risk factor modification programmes, or on 'leader/ development models' encouraging group and community empowerment through raising critical consciousness (Connolly and Emmel forthcoming). In other words, focus is either on biomedical discourses of causation, or on discourses of social location. In the former, the pathology is part of the body and in that sense is part of the individual's life, and to some extent the individual entails taking responsibility for the condition by contributing to it through 'risky practices'. In the latter, a more socio-ecological approach with broader health economics' theories contextualise the individual in a particular socio-historical framework (Braathen 1996: 153), attributing particular socio-demographic features – class, income, ethnicity, gender, location – as having significant impact on an individual's health which have to be dealt with through broader community-wide health initiatives. The consequences of this tension is that a dualism in the individual's identity is implied; individuals are both subject to social circumstances and therefore attention must be given to redressing a lack of agency or, conversely, they have primary responsibility and unimpaired agency and should be taught not to engage in damaging practices.

This tension reflects that imbricated in the discursive constitution of the 'individual' in both CAM and bio-medical encounters, which involve differing conceptualisations of the body, the individual, pathology and the responsibilities accruing to the differentiated roles of patient/user/client in these different care settings and encounters (Mitchell and Cormack 1998). Specifically, 'normative rights' (Sevenhuijsen 2000) such as patient empowerment, autonomy and control in discourses underpinning CAMs, are held to be absent from medical encounters in orthodox medicine. Rather, biomedicine is understood to comprise discourses of pathological bodies worked upon by medical practices where the 'individual-as-self' is absent from such discursive constitutions. Biomedical discourses, it is argued, seek to homogenise bodies and pathologies both in their 'gaze' and their approaches to treatment (see Foucault 1975). Consequently, the biomedical 'individual' (Foucault 1990) is discursively conflated with 'the patient', whose responsibilities, power and authority are circumscribed by their location in the medical setting/encounter, and defined in large part by their lack of scientific medical knowledge and expertise. The individual as patient is therefore subject to medical power and control and thus is perceived as being unable to exercise autonomy (Foucault 1975). Therefore, the individual-as-self, the patient, is conceptually separated from their body which becomes the focus of the medical encounter. In turn, the body is reduced to a pathology, and the individual-as-self is no longer an expert on themselves. Instead, in the medical encounter, their knowledge is 'lay' knowledge and so is lacking constitutive power.

In contrast, many philosophies underpinning CAM consider the pathology to be the pathology of the whole organism (Hahnemann 1986) and so do not entail any ostensible ontological divide between *self* and *body*. CAM practitioners in both studies stated uniformly that they treat the individual, not the disease. By approaching the individual holistically, it was argued, the individual is constituted as combining mind, body, spirit and social location, where both pathology, and therefore treatment, must be unique to that individual. The condition cannot be separated from who and what the individual is. Individuality both of pathology and treatment is therefore central across most CAM philosophies and healing approaches. It is, then, the responsibility of the individual and the CAM practitioner to explore the pathology and, in order to do so, the individual becomes as much an 'expert' as the practitioner (Sharma 1992) and diagnosis is predicated on a full conceptualisation of the individual. As part of this, the patient/user/client is expected to invest not only in the diagnostic process but also the healing process (discussed more fully below), which involves empowering the patient/user/client in the management of their own healthcare. In effect, discourses of CAMs are underpinned by notions of power equality, where practitioner and user come to the therapeutic encounter with their different expertise and both invest in the recovery and health of the user (Mitchell and Cormack 1998).[2]

To these different modes of expertise accrue different responsibilities relating to the individual's process through treatment. The relationship is conceived of as a partnership, thus avoiding power inequalities such as those perceived in relationships patients have with their doctors. The patient's/user's/client's treatment is conceived of as a 'process' or 'pathway' through treatment. It is on this intersection of empowering the patient/user/client, making them responsible for specific healthcare decisions and, to an extent, healthcare provision, that this next section (which forms the bulk of the chapter) will focus, drawing on the empirical data from the two studies mentioned previously.

Ways of being responsible

Seeking treatment and participation in treatment

From analyses of the interviews with CAM practitioners and CAM patients/users/clients, a central tension around the types and extent of the patient's/user's/client's responsibility for ill health emerged, echoing the earlier tension in orthodox medicine and contemporary state discourses of public health. Specifically, patients/users/clients were understood, and understood themselves to be, centrally implicated both in their own health maintenance and their illnesses, yet the extent to which this was the case was frequently negotiated.

Ultimately, the philosophy is about you choose whether you're ill or not. But that's far too big to say to anybody and it sounds like blaming, and sounds like if you're not getting better it's your own fault, which it's not that.

(Massage therapist)

what's different about it [complementary therapy] is that it requests the participation of the patient in a very big way. What it does say, actually why you're ill might be in your hands.

(TCM practitioner)

I'd try not to get in the same state that I was in but a lot of the state I was in was due to things that I had no control over and I could see when the doctor said, well you know, those people have one problem, you know. So I didn't feel quite as guilty. And so some of those problems have gone now and so I really want to get in control again and I would probably go to a homeopathic doctor before it got into the state it got into this last time.

(Patient: CAM homeopathy)

From the interviews it emerged that the patient/user/client was constituted as being responsible for their illness. The extent of this responsibility, however, was unclear and, while it was stated that the causes of illness were negotiated, in the therapy sessions the patient/user/client was, as part of their life, involved in choosing between health and illness. Rather than in some blasé, devil-may-care behaviour on the part of the patient/user/client, resulting in ill health which they could have foreseen, the 'causes' of ill health were clearly embedded in lifestyle behaviours, for example poor diet and lack of exercise, and taking a particular emotional stance on one's life in order to relieve stress. In this way, responsibility was diffused from the individual to their life-, or socio-historical, context. In several of the interviews it emerged that the 'success' of the therapy was negotiated between patient/user/client and CAM practitioner (see below), and that on some occasions this was discussed in the context of the relative responsibilities accruing to the condition, therapy, therapist and/or patient/user/client.

I need to have enough trust with the person [CAM practitioner] to be able to discuss it and to be able to understand what can I do, am I doing something wrong and is it my fault or is it just one of those things. But also it may be that because everybody else says to me 'You've been doing this a long time, why, why aren't you getting better?'

(Patient: GP acupuncture; received homeopathy and osteopathy previously)

However, many patients/users/clients had chosen CAM precisely because doctors considered they were responsible themselves for certain of their conditions, particularly where the condition was considered to some extent to be psychosomatic. In particular, mental illness was framed within a bio-medical discourse that came into conflict with therapeutic/psychological discourses in biomedical encounters. Whilst on the one hand the doctor was implying the patient's behaviour was to some extent the cause of the condition, they were simultaneously reframing the 'cure' as pharmaco-logical rather than therapeutic. In other words, the discourses at play both insisted on and yet removed the patient's agency.

> the [complementary] consultant was very sympathetic, he did not blame me for inflicting it [eczema] on myself which I found mainstream medi-cine did. The doctor sort of wanted me on Valium and Librium and things like that.
>
> (Patient: homeopathy, cranio-sacral therapy, herbalism)

This patient, constantly encouraged to take particular medical drugs to which she was averse, expressed responsibility for the condition both in its genesis and in her lack of compliance with prescribed treatment, to which she had clearly indicated she did not consent. It was at this point that she sought out CAM and that represented a change in her perception of her own efficacy and participation in her own healthcare. This experience was reflected in many of the other interviews with people using CAMs in their departure from orthodox medicine. This process of *seeking out* healthcare in the context of responsibility for one's health, ill health and recovery has been imbued with a range of meanings and responsibilities in both CAM and the NHS (discussed below).

> I don't know whether it's true of all doctors, but certainly the doctors that I've had in the past have not wanted me to know anything about myself and that has been irritating. They've wanted to be able to tell me from a position of superiority and training, which is fine . . . that's why you go to them, you want them to know more than you and be able to do something but I don't want to be out of the equation.
>
> (Massage therapist)

Opportunities for 'control' and 'authority' for the patient/user/client have been identified by CAM users as key reasons for seeking these medicines[3] (Sharma 1992). Users seek out CAM as actively as they seek out treatment on the NHS. As mentioned previously, users of CAMs in our studies felt that seeking out alternative treatment signified a crucial moment of devia-tion from conventional medical care and was retrospectively construed as their initial participation in CAM treatment. CAM practitioners suggested that self-referring clients were more likely to be knowledgeable about the therapy, as opposed to those sent to them from local GP surgeries commissioning a specific number of packages of CAM care. Further, it was felt that 'self-selecting patients are more motivated' and that 'referred patients are not convinced it works' (acupuncturist and TCM practitioner). Complementary therapists in both studies commented that self-selecting, paying patients/users/clients had *already* invested in the process, and were engaged in their own self-care (see also Sharma 1992) and, in this way, contrasted with referred patients from NHS doctors. This latter group of patients, according to the CAM practitioners, were dubious about the effectiveness of the complementary therapy, and it seemed more common for them to state that 'nothing could help' them. These individuals were considered as having already 'failed the process', and all the therapists mentioning this group stated a future intention of telling the individual not to waste the therapist's and their own time.[4] The third group was identified by the CAM practitioners working with people with HIV/AIDS, who suggested that non-paying patients/users/clients were more likely to skip sessions, or to not follow advice. By not paying, CAM practitioners suggested they were less likely to see themselves as *already* having invested in the process. The patients/users/clients of these practitioners, however, stated that the therapies involved a lot of time, physical mobility and mental space in their lives. This enhanced their perceptions of themselves as actively participating in their own healthcare. Further, the suggestion that not paying led to a lack of investment in the therapy did not reflect the perceptions of patients in the local health authority study.

> Q. You mentioned something earlier about paying. Do you think that does make a difference to the way you approach the therapy or the treatment?
> A. Not particularly, because as I say when I was going to the doctors I used to pay to go to the specialist, I had to pay for the blood test, I had to pay for the radiotherapy. I had to pay for the treatment, which was not available on the NHS. My own GP had not even heard of some of the treatment I was having. So all my prescriptions were coming through via the specialist passed up to the GP – so I was paying them. So I can't say that 'Oh, I trust the homoeopath because I have paid for her, so I am buying her time to give me attention'. I also pay the specialist, I also buy my medication – but I don't have the same kind of trust.
> (Patient: homoeopathy, cranio-sacral therapy, herbalism)

In other words, the effort in terms of time, geographical mobility, uniqueness of treatment and financial investment were considered by a number of the patients/users/clients to be similar in both CAM and NHS healthcare settings. The difference lay in terms of the quality of the relationship they developed with the CAM practitioner as opposed to that with their GP, of whom it was, unsurprisingly, said that he/she did not have enough time to invest in the doctor–patient relationship.

Working out what is wrong: is this illness me or not?

Earlier in this chapter, the nature of the 'individual' in the context of both biomedical and CAM discourses was discussed, where the individual was constituted as a patient through biomedical discourse and in state discourses as a participative partner (see also below); whereas the individual in discourses of CAM apparently lacked the ontological separation of mind/self and body inherent in an episteme of health based on biomedical discourse. However, when the mechanisms by which CAM works, or the principles upon which it works as described in the interviews, were explored in more depth it was apparent that these explanations also entailed the separation of mind/self from body. Indeed, the body in some CAM discourse appeared to gain a 'mind' of its own. I will now consider the ways in which the CAM practitioners described their therapy as working in the context of considerations of the responsibilities individuals accrue in the process of their healthcare.

The responsibility of the individual in CAM therapy

In all the interviews CAMs were presented as an ongoing process entailing a processual relationship into which both the practitioner and patient/user/ client enter, and where both participate in the task of encouraging the patient's/user's/client's body to self-heal (see below; see also Mitchell and Cormack 1998). This is predicated on an understanding of the individuality of both the practitioner and patient/user/client where they are in a constant state of change. The practitioner engages with the patient/user/client on the understanding that they are not necessarily the same as they were in the previous session, particularly as attitude change is considered to be an important and desired outcome of therapy. The practitioners themselves, through practising their therapy, are also in some slight way altered. Additionally, a significant proportion of the practitioners interviewed indicated that therapy was a processual relationship between therapist and patient/user/client and what occurs *between* the therapist and patient/user/ client is of an ongoing nature.

> sometimes I consider some of the successful practitioner–patient relationships that I have to be not based on reduction in headaches, but helping somebody through witnessing their process.
>
> (Acupuncturist and TCM practitioner)

Thus, to some extent, the therapeutic intervention is understood as being less engaged in 'curing' the condition and more in guiding the patient/user/client through 'change'. CAMs, engaged in changing the individual as part of the healing process, can be understood as both means and ends, rather than just a means to an end – a concept frequently juxtaposed with perceptions of conventional medicine in the interviews with both practitioners and patients/users/clients. A particular feature of this process, particularly in the 'touch therapies' (massage, reflexology, shiatsu, aromatherapy), is that treating and touching the patient/user/client is both treatment and further diagnosis. Treatment becomes an exploration, which seeks to further inform the therapist of the patient's/user's/client's body. Therefore, unlike biomedicine, which aims to deal with the specific condition/symptom presented in the initial consultation session with the patient/user/client and to treat only that until it is gone, CAM practitioners expect their therapies to *reveal* further conditions and complaints, which they will diagnose and treat on an ongoing basis. This process of learning more about the patient's/user's/client's body is undertaken by both the practitioner and the patient/user/client, the latter actively encouraged to learn and be open to this learning process as part of their treatment.

Many CAM therapies are considered to work on a number of levels and part of this philosophy is that the condition is often not merely physical. This is not always necessarily the case but, throughout the interviews, the case histories cited commonly suggested that the condition worked on a number of levels. It was argued that the condition embodied an emotional statement: '[that's] what eczema is, keep out, I don't want anyone getting in there' (massage therapist) and was 'a signal of something else going on' (yoga therapist). Further, that the body had a 'mind' of its own, articulated through symptoms, some of which were more important than others. Indeed, the condition itself was considered descriptive of the patient/user/client presenting with it, with symptoms as the expression of a person's attempts to heal themself (homeopath).

Therefore the self-healing mechanisms by which people recover require the individual's input either psychologically or physically, whether or not they use CAM or biomedical treatments (see below). Importantly, this learning process entails relearning ways of experiencing embodiment. One osteopath argued that it is the individual's perception of pain that guides their behaviour and influences their experience of their condition.[5] Both the osteopaths interviewed for the local health authority study argued that pain is not an adequate indicator of the individual's condition. Instead, pain is subjective, in that one person's severe pain may be another person's mild pain, changing over time. Indeed, it was argued in these interviews that changes in the individual's neural network, where experiences of pain are *accommodated* and incorporated in the individual's experience of embodiment, may result in them experiencing continuing pain when there ought to be none, any underlying pathology having disappeared. In other words, the body becomes habituated to certain physical states. CAM practitioners interviewed stated that the majority of their patients/users/clients usually suffer from chronic rather than acute conditions, and were likely to be deeply embedded in practices contributing to their ill health. Thus both 'body' and 'individual', discursively constituted as separate, could be considered as requiring re-education. Re-educating the individual involved not only the appropriate physical changes they should make in their lives (for example, more exercise), but also their perceptions of pain. In the case of osteopathy, the body and the 'mind' were considered to be re-educated both in understanding and communicating with each other, as part of the individual's education in practical techniques of self-care.[6]

This also emerged in talk about the responsibility of the patient/user/ client in terms of their engagement with the healing process, beyond behaviour and lifestyle modification. Many CAM practitioners emphasised that the practitioner–client relationship involved negotiation about what needed to be treated first, or most urgently, and negotiations centred on perceived need and professional diagnosis. Although the patient/user/client may not know what *needs* to be treated first, their ideas about what they *want* to be treated informed the CAM practitioner about the type of person they were and, in turn, informed treatment and diagnosis:

> I would say well, why would you want to deal with that first? . . . It may be important to finding out about the person. But what the person says is important to what I might prescribe. What they want is different from, what their perception of what they need is something different, quite often different, from what the practitioner believes they need. . . . If they have a problem which they perceive is affecting their life so much then that obviously needs to be looked at very closely. That's the point at which if they're the strongest symptoms at the time, that's the body saying, well this situation needs to be dealt with because it could be life threatening at its most extreme.
>
> (Homeopath)

This statement is predicated on similar discursive constitutions of the practitioner as expert, as 'meta-listening' and (re)formulating the patient's problem (Davis 1986) according to the practitioner's expertise. Whilst this cannot be taken as representative of all homeopaths, or indeed CAM practitioners, in a number of interviews this discursive constitution of 'expert' and 'lay' occurred. Importantly, here, the body is again presented as 'speaking' to the therapist through its symptoms, and in this way speaking to the individual-as-self, as ontologically separate. Whilst in this example, in contrast to that given by the osteopaths, the body is capable of speaking an inner 'truth' (it is reliable); it is the body that is to be listened to. In this sense, the discursive constitution of the body, the self and the practitioner-as-expert all work towards blurring the boundaries of the domain of responsibility and, in some of the interviews, was expressed as a confusion around the sort of investment in recovery the patient/user/client should be making.

Taking time

Time, a constant criticism of biomedicine/NHS healthcare, in the context of the individual's engagement in the recovery process was perceived as dependent on the 'contract' between the patient/user/client and CAM practitioner. Paying for one's treatment meant that the time spent belongs to the person that is paying and, as mentioned previously, the CAM practitioners considered that paying for the treatment formalises the commitment of the patient/user/client to their own self-healing, an integral part of the self-healing process.

Having faith

In addition to compliance, lifestyle and behaviour changes and changes in self and body perception, patients/users/clients are responsible for belief and confidence in treatment. A key difference between CAMs and NHS health-care concerned perceptions of CAM therapy as 'faith healing'. Whilst this was an avowed component of many CAM therapies, according to the practitioners interviewed for our studies, it was perceived to be a silent, disavowed yet integral component of orthodox medical treatment: 'if one is to talk about faith healing, there's more faith in doctors than in CAM practitioners' (massage therapist). However, CAMs are defined as an 'alternative' set of practices and philosophies of health and healing in the context of biomedical discourses, where biomedicine is a self-legitimating set of medical practices and discourses with a particular orientation towards the body (Foucault 1975); CAMs require conscious belief on the part of the patient/user/client that they are going to work. In contrast, patients/users/clients are perceived to be uncritical of the scientific *basis* of biomedicine, and unlikely to criticise the efficacy of biomedicine as a scientific discipline. Indeed, it was considered by some CAM practitioners interviewed that belief in conventional medicine may affect the rapidity of the healing process. In the context of their own therapies, as part of belief and faith, almost all practitioners stated that the patient/user/client must want to get better and be open to the treatment: 'do people have to allow this to happen to them? Yes, they do. Anybody, whatever medicine you're taking, has to empower the process' (acupuncturist and TCM practitioner).

As with biomedicine, it was argued, the intention of the patient/user/client using CAMs to get better affects the degree of success of the healing process, and negative expectations retard or inhibit the healing process. Therefore, in large part, the patient/user/client must intend to have a powerful experience of change, essential to any medical intervention.

Success of the treatment

Some CAM practitioners considered expectations of success were different between biomedicine and CAM, in that 'biomedicine isn't considered successful unless the condition's gone and it stays gone' (massage therapist). Defining 'health', 'illness' and 'recovery' is a process in which both patient/user/client and practitioner are involved in CAM and where the patient/user/client has responsibilities in participating in the ongoing diagnostic process, developing criteria for success of treatment in synchrony with the CAM practitioner and negotiating around definitions of 'health', which do not necessarily relate to those used in other medical models. Further, that overall responsibility for health is the individual's, both in everyday life and in treatment sessions, even though they may attempt to hand over responsibility for their ill health to the CAM practitioner. Nevertheless, when patients/users/clients take responsibility for their own health this may be considered a sign of success and, indeed, enhance the treatment.

Avoiding blame

However, where this is the case, the patient/user/client must also assume responsibility for the treatment not working, as psychological as well as active physical compliance is entailed. Overall, success was largely defined as the acquisition of self-knowledge by the patient/user/client, and this occurred at the point at which the individual could maintain the change they experienced, and continue to maintain it over a long period of time. Reasons for therapy not working included an unwillingness on the part of the patient/user/client to change or get better by letting go of their condition because, perhaps, it was part of the way they lived and may be one mechanism with which they negotiate their social relationships. Alternatively, they may still have been doing something that was producing the problem, or the wrong diagnosis had been made. Further, it may be that there was very serious pathology and that, perhaps, it was too late for any treatment to work. It is important at this juncture to include a statement by one of the CAM practitioners who pointed out that in some cases, such as with cancer or HIV, the individual could be considered as having had 'their franchise taken away'. The implication of this was that first, it was inappropriate to blame the individual, and second that although they should still participate in their health maintenance, the potency of their condition established the boundaries and limitations of their own and others' effectiveness. Whilst CAM practitioners wish to overcome the perceived, artificial separation of person from body and emotions from physical state, where one can be seen as imbricated in the other, it is inappropriate and inaccurate to *blame* the individual for being ill. Nevertheless, for some of the patients/users/clients, the sense of 'guilt' impinged on their perceptions of self-efficacy in their healthcare.

When to end treatment

A concern mentioned by the CAM practitioners was to balance the health of the patient/user/client (how much pain they could live with, how skilled they became at health management and maintenance, how sophisticated their attitudes to their health had become) with the danger of their becoming a 'therapy junkie'. That is, one aspect of the practitioners' role was to decide how long the patient/user/client should participate in therapy. The end of the therapy relationship is negotiated between the practitioner and patient/user/client, who ought to cease therapy when they no longer need it and could take sole responsibility for their own health maintenance. Therefore, 'health' becomes 'healthy enough', a matter of negotiation rather than a given physical state. Although still suffering from particular pains and conditions, it was apparently quite common for people to stop therapy as they were (as a consequence of the CAM therapy) now engaged in a process of *self-maintenance* rather than in a search for a 'cure'. Whilst there is a great deal of debate about the inclusion criteria of the term 'health' (Lowenberg and Davis 1994), it is possible to assume that it is to do with 'the lack of a disease process'. Instead, health (and ill health) is more to do with aspects of the individual's ability in areas such as emotional and mental balance, interpretations of physical state and physical pain, and the somatisation of emotional distress.

In summary, the individual becomes implicated, again, in their own (ill)health. Rather than something happening to them, they, either through an inherited constitution, through inadequate health maintenance habits and behaviour (stated all the practitioners interviewed) or, particularly through stress, participate to some degree in their ill health, or lack of good health. 'Empowering the process' means encouraging the patients/users/clients' contribution to, and investment in, their own healing process. This might involve belief in the effectiveness of the therapy, changing behaviour to support the therapy, attending the therapist in the first place (thus signifying an intention to improve their condition), and making a commitment to ongoing change in their lives. For CAM practitioners interviewed, the intention is that the patient/user/client is empowered through knowledge, training, the experiences of egalitarian participation in their own healthcare and their commitment to their ongoing health maintenance. The patient/user/client is constituted as responsible for initiating the treatment, engaging in the treatment, engaging in improving health either through self-care or belief, in negotiating definitions of success and, finally, for ending the therapeutic process with the CAM practitioner. In this way, the responsibility for the patient's/user's/client's healthcare is discursively shifted from the practitioner in CAMs to the patient/user/client, where what is 'healthy' is presented as the 'individual' engaged healthily in their life-context.

The role of the individual in NHS healthcare

It is useful at this juncture to reconsider the biomedical context in which CAMs operate. As mentioned, in biomedical discourses what is presented is the condition, and the individual/patient is reduced to a vehicle for the pathology (Martin 1987). Whilst this may be a central tenet of biomedical discourse, it is however useful to shift our focus from the systems of knowledge describing the mechanisms of biomedicine to the processes of healthcare. In doing so, it becomes clear that the patient re-emerges as capable of agency. Indeed, the UK state's description of the techniques currently available to them as part of their engagement in their healthcare in the UK NHS necessitates a reconceptualisation of the patient as accruing particular rights and responsibilities (Dyke 1998). Although much literature on the doctor–patient relationship explicates the ways in which partnership is impossible because of the entrenched knowledge/power differentials (Fisher and Groce 1985), this has nevertheless become a dominant theme in recent manifestos outlining what patients ought to be able to expect from their doctors. Indeed, it is on the basis of partnership that the patient has been rewritten into medical encounters in the NHS (see below). It is, then, inadequate to reduce discourses of the patient to biomedical discourses of bodily pathology. Rather, it is more useful to consider biomedical discourse in the context of UK state debates around health and illness and the patient's journey from one to the other through particular care settings and treatments. As with CAMs, increasingly in the NHS, the patient's treatment is conceived of as a process or pathway through treatment. It is this intersection of empowering the patient, making them responsible for specific healthcare decisions and, to an extent, healthcare provision in both the NHS and in CAMs that the rest of this chapter will focus. The following discussion will explore the different responsibilities accruing at each stage of the patient's process through treatment: becoming ill, seeking treatment, what the treatment does, recovery, success and ending the treatment.

> Because the NHS is trying to educate people now more about health and how to be more preventative, and looking at more preventative medicine, but in fact, the whole premise of where the medicine is, looking at the illness and dissecting illness, knowing about illness and the

one virus that causes the problem. Whereas health is more than that and there is no concept of health in Western medicine.

(Acupuncturist)

This quotation admirably summarises a large part of the medicalisation debate (Fox 1993) where the individual becomes a patient as soon as they enter the health service, regardless of the reason for which they consult healthcare services. In UK state discourse on the role of the patient, the focus is on rights, responsibilities and participation. The remainder of this chapter will concentrate on the specific features of these in the context of the preceding discussion of the patient's responsibilities in CAMs.

Much health promotion work has focused on ways of educating the individual, looking at information provision, at ways of most effectively contextualising information, at who provides information and how information can be presented in such a way that the individual has ongoing access to the meanings provided. It is precisely this tension that emerges in state discourses of self-care and preventive care – the 'frontline' in any individual engagement in healthcare practices – and is reflected in emerging expectations of patients' responsibilities in caring for themselves, preventing illness and seeking out treatment. UK state definitions of self-care involve social definitions of care reliant on caregiving, as part of familial roles, care as an ethic or moral orientation supporting the welfare of the collectivity, and care as work (Daly forthcoming). As the *NHS Plan* (2000) outlines:

> The frontline in healthcare is the home. Most healthcare starts with people looking after themselves and their families at home. The NHS will become a resource which people routinely use every day to help look after themselves. 0845 46 47 will become one of the best-used phone numbers as millions of people every year contact NHS Direct to get advice about health problems. Each week will see millions of hits on the NHS Direct internet site. As well as providing fast and reliable information on a wide range of conditions, it will also be valued as an easy way to contact patient and self-help groups.

Self-care in state discourse therefore involves the patient (already a patient *before* they access services) using technologies which include the internet, digital TV and NHSplus and, supported by healthcare professionals, trained in self-care, particularly for chronic conditions (*NHS Plan* 2000). Patients are thus encouraged to exercise authority, control and autonomy around accessing services and managing ongoing conditions. Effectively, the 'expert patient' becomes the primary commissioner of healthcare, involved in organising and tailoring healthcare services to their perceived needs.

This is not dissimilar to central tenets of CAM philosophy around the re-education and training elements of CAM therapy. Importantly, in the area of information provision and *retention and understanding,* the patient's responsibilities and rights are most clearly stressed. Indeed, the patient now becomes the expert patient, provided with patient-friendly versions of clinical guidelines from the National Institute for Clinical Excellence (NICE), and with greater information about treatment planned for them and access to their medical records. Effectively, the patient is encouraged to become a proactive leader in the commissioning of healthcare services for their self-perceived needs, and potential entry points into healthcare services are redesigned in order to facilitate access by the patient.

In this context, preventive care emerges as a series of pre-emptive strikes against potential illness and disease. As participative citizens in the NHS, patients are encouraged to participate in routine screening which, it has been suggested, will be extended to cover more conditions in order to mini-mise the risks to their health, using conventional tests or the new genetic tests. In the context of public health education, as treatments such as these are becoming increasingly available, it is interesting to consider the extent to which patients can become expert in routine screening and decide whether there are alternatives, either of screening processes or different epistemes of an individual's responsibility in their self-care. Care innova-tions such as these beg ethical questions around informed consent and, indeed, around informed refusal to consent. Additionally, patients will be offered advice on diet and exercise as part of a routine service at their local surgery and, where registers are kept in areas where ill health is most preva-lent, people may be offered preventive treatment. 'Underlying causes of ill health' are therefore simultaneously defined both in terms of individual behaviour and in the context of local prevalence of particular conditions. In other words, UK state discourse is beginning to reflect CAM philosophy which, for so long, has insisted on perceiving the individual as already socially located and engaged in particular (un)healthy practices.

In support of these initiatives, patient choice emerges as a strong theme in UK state discourse, where the patient accrues a set of rights around choos-ing their GP as part of exercising informed choice based on information published about each GP. As part of this, patients will have the right to access an advocate, that is, an independent facilitator handling patient and family concerns to ensure support for the people complaining. In other words, the patient gains rights to a professional voice within the NHS, a voice by proxy. It is clear that in UK state discourses around participation and responsibility in healthcare, the potential for success of treatment is primarily based on the patient making themselves available (seeking diag-nosis) early enough in the course of their ill-health. In effect, as a partici-pative citizen of the NHS, patients become technologically competent, geographically mobile (able to attend centres of excellence nationwide), self-diagnosing and self-referring (going to one-stop centres). Therefore, in *contacting* the NHS they become the commissioning partner: however, once involved in care services their commissioning partner is their GP and their responsibility is to give informed consent (that is, they have to say if they don't understand).[7]

Importantly, it is the nature of the patient-as-individual which has been implicated in a number of recent historical changes and negotiations in UK government statements and manifestos pointing to responsibilities and rights in the NHS (for example, *Patients Charter, NHS Charter, NHS Plan*). Historically, the NHS has been represented as a marketplace in order to enhance internal effectiveness by drawing on what have been seen as the lessons from and strengths of the private sector. Here, the patient has been defined as a customer (Freidson 1970; Silverman 1983) or consumer of services. The limitations of this discursive constitution of the patient, in terms of their access to power and their opportunities for exercising power and control, have elsewhere been documented (Taylor 1985). Specifically, the power differentials inherent in the power–knowledge nexus of the medical encounter (Foucault 1990) ensure it is not enough for a patient to exhibit lay expertise nor, indeed, any medical expertise; some medical practitioners consider that patients should be given information by their doctor rather than seeking information for themselves (Dyke 1998). Instead, it is necessary for the NHS as a complex nexus of relationships and services, underpinned by particular normative frameworks (Sevenhuijsen 2000), to both safeguard patients' rights and empower the patient throughout their progress through their healthcare (*NHS Plan* 2000). Thus, the healthcare process for the patient through the NHS care setting is one whereby disempowerment through lack of professional knowledge is redressed through the attribution of rights[8] and a systemic orientation towards the patient is driven by values of empowerment through information, support and involvement. In other words or, more specifically in the words of CAM practitioners, *empowering the process*. What empowerment means in UK state discourses as being anything beyond being informed, with (prescribed) choices of services and with right of redress, is yet to be revealed.

As the current Labour government develops 'the Third Way' (Giddens 1994), this involvement of the patient in their own healthcare is conceived of in the context of the 'participative citizen' (Sevenhuijsen 2000). Here, citizenship involves participation in all sectors of society in which the individual operates or acts, both formally and informally. To assume the responsibilities and duties of a citizen is to participate in all aspects of social life in which one is involved. In the healthcare setting, 'the patient and/or the person responsible for them' have been charged with the task of 'working in partnership' (*NHS Plan* 2000) with the healthcare professionals with whom they come in contact. Thus, practices of engagement in social-sector settings are simultaneously practices of participative citizenship necessary for authenticity and legitimacy in the role of citizen-patient. The *NHS Plan* (2000) can be read as a manifesto of the duties and responsibilities of patients and carers in all healthcare settings. In the context of the Patient's Charter (1992) and the proposed NHS Charter (Dyke 1998), where the *rights* of the patient and carer have been defined in order to rectify perceived entrenched power inequalities in the doctor–patient relationship, the discourses used and interventions suggested ostensibly rectify any power imbalance in favour of the patient and carer or any users of healthcare services. Additionally, by linking up the responsibilities and duties of patients, carers and practitioners in healthcare engagement and practices, the participative patient becomes an informal 'worker', and it is precisely in terms of 'work' that the patient's responsibilities in the NHS are described.

This participative role is both formal and informal. The patient-citizen is encouraged to participate at a number of levels in feeding information and views to the NHS (for example, positions on the General Medical Council, the new Modernisation Board, the new Independent Reconfiguration Panel on contested major service changes, the review teams for the Commission for Health Improvement and a new Citizens Council to advise the National Institute for Clinical Excellence on its clinical assessments). Thus, the patient-citizen will inform the process by which patient information is produced. The implications of this are that the patient-citizen, or a specific number of patient-citizens, are to be involved in the ongoing organisation and orientation of patient-centred (and patient empowered) healthcare services.

Conclusion

Earlier in this chapter it was argued that seeking healthcare and being involved in healthcare significantly contributes to the processes of identity constitution in which people are engaged. If we consider the different explanations offered by CAMs and biomedicine to explain the mechanisms by which their respective interventions actually work, it would be possible to expect each approach to differently constitute the patient. However, by using a discourse analytic approach, shifting our focus from technologies of healing to the processes of healthcare facilitates a meaningful comparison of the ways in which the individual is imbued with and accrues a series of responsibilities for their healthcare in conventional medicine and CAMs. Self-care emerges as an inherently social activity, linking not only the individual's intra-local domains, but also drawing together activities connecting individual, state and society (Daly 2002). Even prior to entering primary care, individuals are constituted within state discourse as being responsible for particular self-care practices and are defined as *working with* the NHS. Within CAM philosophy, the patient's/user's/client's responsibilities are clearly similar: they are responsible for maintaining their health and seeking appropriate healthcare when they are beset with ill health, and this is part of self-care. Central tensions for each approach around the extent of the patient's/user's/client's responsibility emerge simultaneously with this micro/macro relationship: how far are they or their socio-historical context responsible for their ill-health, for their ability appropriately to seek health-care, and for their ability to learn new healthier self-care techniques? Specifically, CAM practitioners and patients express a sense of struggle with stopping *responsibility* from collapsing into *blame*. The analyses presented in this chapter suggest that both in CAM and biomedical explanations of how their treatment works and the processes of healthcare in which they engage with the patient/user/client, there is a conflation and confusion of the discourses of causation and discourses of social location. The individual is approached holistically and yet their body speaks with a distinct and separate voice through symptoms and pathology. Similarly, therapeutic and biomedical discourses converge on the CAM practitioner–client encounter, introducing tensions around issues of expertise and authority (particularly around the extent to which the body speaks more truthfully than the patient).

In conclusion, it is clear that simplistic distinctions between conventional medicine and CAM fail to provide the opportunity for analysis of the socio-historical location and development of different epistemes of health and healing.

Notes

1 As I will be exploring the roles and responsibilities of individuals in different healthcare settings, when I refer to biomedicine I am talking specifically in the context of the UK NHS. My argument, in part, will focus on the constitution of the political, socio-economic role of the individual as patient in this and in CAM healthcare settings.

2 Further, that the patient is 'empowered' through the course of their therapy.

3 Could be useful in making sense of the development of CAM as a process of healthcare in the Western world.

4 This point refers specifically to the need for the patient/user/client to 'invest in the treatment', which is discussed more fully later.

5 This was particularly so in the context of back pain, especially low back pain, where common practice is to 'lay up', conserving the back, whereas medical evidence points to the efficacy of continued activity and that conserving the back may well contribute to the condition.

6 This was also a theme raised in the context of CAMs encouraging the body to 'forget' or 'recover from' ancient injuries or illnesses which it was in some way holding onto. In these interviews, the body was distinctly constituted as having

a 'mind of its own', this being a verbatim expression of a number of practitioners and one patient.

7 It is very tempting to argue on the basis of this position-statement that patients are understood to be consenting as long as they are not complaining.

8 However, these rights have been described as 'quasi-rights', boiling down to the rights of the patient to complain if the quality of service, treatment or care falls below the standards outlined in the emerging National Service Frameworks (NSFs) (Dyke 1998).

References

Banister, P., Burman, E., Parker, I., Taylor, M. and Tindall, C. (1995) *Qualitative Methods in Psychology: a research guide*, Buckingham: Open University Press.

Bordo, S. (1995) *Unbearable Weight: feminism, Western culture and the body*, London: University of California Press.

Braathen, E., (1996) 'Communicating the individual body and the body politic: the discourse on disease prevention and health promotion in alternative therapies', in Cant, S. and Sharma, U. (eds), *Complementary and Alternative Medicines: knowledge in practice*, London: Free Association Books.

Connolly, J. and Emmel, N.D. (forthcoming) *Preventing Disease or Helping the Struggle for Participation: does professional public health have a future?* Policy and Politics.

Coward, R. (1989) *The Whole Truth: the myth of alternative health*, London: Faber & Faber.

Daly, M. (forthcoming) 'Care as a good for social policy', *Journal of Social Policy*.

Davis, K., (1986) 'The process of problem (re)formulation in psychotherapy', *Sociology of Health and Illness* 8,1: 44–74.

Dyke, G. (1998) *The New NHS charter: a different approach*. Online. Available HTTP:
http://www.doh.gov.uk/pub/docs/doh/dyke.pdf

Elias, N. (1978) *The Civilising Process, vol. 1, The History of Manners*, Oxford: Basil Blackwell.

Ehrenreich, B. and English, D. (1988) *For Her Own Good. 150 years of the expert's advice to women*, London: Pluto.

Fisher, S. and Groce, S.B. (1985) 'Doctor–patient negotiation of cultural assumptions', *Sociology of Health and Illness* 7,3: 342–74.

Foucault, M. (1972), *History of Sexuality, vol. 1*, Harmondsworth: Penguin.

Foucault, M. (1975) *The Birth of the Clinic: an archaeology of medical perception*, New York: Vintage Books.

Foucault, M. (1990) *The History of Sexuality: The care of the self, vol. 3*, Harmondsworth: Penguin.

Fox, N.J. (1993) *Postmodernism, Sociology and Health*, Philadelphia: OUP Buckingham.

Freidson, E. (1970) *Professional Dominance*, Chicago: Atherton Press.

Giddens, A. (1994) *Beyond Left and Right*, Cambridge: Polity Press.

Hahnemann, S. (1986) *Organon of Medicine*, New Delhi: B. Jain.

Hughes, K., Long, A., Mercer, G., Ruddlesden, J. and Worth, C. (1997) *Developing and Piloting the Holistic Outcomes Monitoring Tool,* Calderdale & Kirklees Health Authority.

Long, A., Mercer, G. and Hughes, K. (2000) 'Developing a tool to measure holistic practice: a missing dimension in outcomes measurement within complementary therapies', *Complementary Therapies in Medicine* 8: 26–31.

Lowenberg, J.S. and Davis, F. (1994) 'Beyond medicalisation–demedicalisation: the case of holistic health', *Sociology of Health and Illness* 16,5: 579–99.

Martin, E. (1987) *The Woman in the Body*, Milton Keynes: Open University Press.

Mitchell, A. and Cormack, M. (1998) *The Therapeutic Relationship in Complementary Health Care*, London: Churchill Livingstone.

Nettleton, S. (1991) 'Wisdom, diligence and teeth: discursive practices and the creation of mothers', *Sociology of Health and Illness* 13,1: 98–111.

NHS Plan, Department of Health (2000) Online. Available HTTP: http://www.doh.gov.uk/nhsplan/nhsplan.htm

Sevenhuijsen, S. (2000) 'Normative concepts in Dutch policies on work and care', in Bashevkin, S. (ed.) *Women's Work Is Never Done: comparative studies in care-giving, employment and social policy reform.* New York: Routledge.

Sharma, U. (1992) *Complementary Medicine Today: practitioners and patients*, London: Tavistock/Routledge.

Shilling, C. (1993) *The Body and Social Theory*, London: Sage.

Silverman, D. (1983) 'The clinical subject: adolescents in a cleft-palate clinic', *Sociology of Health and Illness* 5,3: 253–74.

Taylor, R. (1985) 'Alternative medicine and the medical encounter in Britain and the United States', in Salmon, J.W. (ed.) *Alternative Medicines: popular and policy perspectives,* London: Tavistock.

Part II

The structural context of the state and the market

Chapter 3

Evidence-based medicine and CAM

Evan Willis and Kevin White

Introduction

This chapter is a sociological analysis of the relationship between two important social movements in healthcare: the continued rise in demand for and patronage of the services of complementary and alternative medicines (CAM) on the one hand, and of evidence-based medicine/health services (EBM) on the other. It concentrates in particular on the implications and challenges of one (EBM) for the other (CAM), utilising the concept of legitimacy as a theoretical tool for analysis of these social processes in the unfolding of healthcare provision in general and in Australian society in particular. First though, it is necessary to review the rise of each of these social movements.

The rise of EBM

At its most basic, evidence-based medicine is claimed to be a methodology for medical decision-making. It was developed at McMaster University in Hamilton, Ontario by a group of epidemiologists who promoted it as a practice of 'integrating individual clinical expertise with the best available external clinical evidence from systematic research' (Sackett *et al*. 1996; see also Sackett *et al*. 1997: 2). The implications of EBM for orthodox medical practice in general have been analysed elsewhere and are far from clear (see Willis and White forthcoming). This chapter focuses on its implications for CAM in particular. The question of whether it constitutes a whole new perspective or paradigm of medical knowledge and practice is a controversial one. Its proponents certainly espouse it to be so, claiming that it is a wholly new form of medical practice (see Guyatt 1993: 10) mostly in the form, on the one hand, of ongoing self-education of practitioners (based on an appraisal of the 'latest' and most objective data available from 'gold standard' double-blind trials and longitudinal studies) and, on the other hand, allowing for patient input in decisions regarding their healthcare. But others disagree (see Rangachari 1997). It is perhaps ironic that Kuhn

(1962) himself excluded medicine from his list of paradigms because there were too many human factors involved.

What EBM actually means for health policy is complex and unresolved at this historical juncture (see Neissen *et al.* 2000). It may mean different things to different stakeholders and in different countries, especially between North America and Europe (see Daly forthcoming). What started out in Canada as aiming to inform clinicians has been used, for instance in the British context, to inform policy-makers. More recently, there has come to be a more consumer-focused element to EBM (Daly forthcoming). Sackett (2000: 1283) has reflected on this changing meaning in a letter to the BMJ. With his tongue firmly planted in his cheek, he identifies '*Sackettisation*' as a new word in medical circles meaning: 'the artificial linkage of a publication to the evidence-based medicine movement in order to improve sales'.

EBM, as a methodology, privileges certain types of evidence over others and arranges these in a hierarchy with randomised controlled trials (preferably of the double-blind crossover variety) at the apex. In this sense, EBM represents a linear historical development from clinical practice guidelines and the Cochrane Collaboration. As adapted for use in the Australian context from an American source (Fisher 1989; NHMRC 1995) this hierarchy of authority is shown in Box 3.1.

Box 3.1 Hierarchy of authority
Level I
Evidence obtained from a systematic review of all relevant randomised controlled trials.
Level II
Evidence obtained from at least one properly designed randomised controlled trial.
Level III.1
Evidence obtained from well-designed controlled trials without randomisation.
Level III.2
Evidence obtained from well-designed cohort or case-control analytic studies, preferably from more than one centre or research group.
Level III.3
Evidence obtained from multiple time series with or without the intervention. Dramatic results in uncontrolled experiments (such as the introduction of penicillin treatment in the 1940s) could also be regarded as this type of evidence.
Level IV
Opinions of respected authorities, based on clinical experience, descriptive studies, or reports of expert committees.

Since its emergence, EBM has now swept across orthodox medicine as its fashionable status has intensified. A largely progressive social movement has emerged as universities have sought to climb aboard this latest of medical bandwagons. Centres and chairs for EBM have been established in many universities and new journals and websites have emerged. EBM has reared its head in unlikely places: in a past Australian federal election the incumbent Minister of Health was heard to castigate his opponents for not having a policy on EBM with which to go to the Australian people. The movement has rubbed off on many other modalities: evidence-based nursing, psychiatry and health management have all appeared. No area of healthcare appears to be immune from catching the evidence-based bug. It is the implications of this social movement for CAM that is the particular focus here.

The rise of CAM

As is documented elsewhere in this book, in a variety of countries and contexts, when ill health strikes, individuals are increasingly consulting non-orthodox practitioners in preference to – or in addition to – 'conventional Western' practitioners (Eisenberg *et al.* 1993; MacLennan *et al.* 1996; Paramore 1997).

Nonetheless, while there does not seem to be much doubt that patronage of CAM is generally increasing, there are some constraints on how certain we can be of the extent of this phenomenon. First, it may just be possible that a substantial proportion of individuals has *always* consulted CAM practitioners: it was just not researched. Or perhaps respondents chose not to reveal to researchers the extent of their patronage of CAM. As many orthodox practitioners have indicated in various research projects, many patients will not reveal what CAM treatments they have been pursuing for fear of their doctor's disapproval. Nonetheless, the evidence does seem to suggest that the increase in the patronage of CAM practitioners is real. Additionally, there is some evidence to suggest that people are *not* so much voting with their feet in turning to CAM practitioners but, rather, the patronage of both orthodox *and* CAM practitioners is increasing (see Astin 1998) – perhaps a plausible explanation as the population ages and chronicity of disease becomes more common.

Second there are problems of definition. CAMs have little in common except for their designation in terms of 'otherness' in relation to the orthodox medical profession. Even a shared holistic approach to CAM is more often expressed as an ideology than as the result of deep adherence (see Berliner and Salmon 1980). Aspects of orthodox medicine can likewise also be considered holistic. The practices of CAM practitioners are based upon many different paradigms of disease and treatment. A recent encyclopedia of modalities reviewed more than 150 (Kastner and Burroughs

1996). As Eisenberg (quoted in Yamey 2000) has claimed, there are 'so many labels, so little consensus'. Indeed, the use of the term 'CAM' in many respects conceals as much as it reveals; it is not overstating the case to say that most CAM modalities have only their ostracism by conventional medicine in common, and even that is a matter of degree.

The underlying basis to these reservations with the now common term of 'complementary and alternative' can be explained further, using insights from the sociology of science. In particular, the issue of commensurability is discussed by Kuhn (1962). Broadly speaking, this concept refers to the extent to which there is translatability between paradigms due to having an integral common measure. By way of example, are the paradigms of allopathy (the historical forerunner of Western scientific biomedicine) and the CAM modality of homeopathy able to be considered commensurable, such that they could be designated complementary? Allopathy is based upon the theory of opposites: that a disease may be cured with a chemical substance that has the opposite therapeutic effect (for example, an anti-biotic). Homeopathy on the other hand, has, as a central plank to its paradigm of healthcare knowledge, the principle that 'like cures like' (see Kaufman 1971). Hence the principal therapeutic tool for homeopaths of preparing medicines by diluting them, from a homeopathic perspective, actually *increases* their potency. From an allopathic perspective however, diluting a chemical substance (often many times to the point where few molecules of the original chemical compound actually remain) *decreases* its potency. In other words, allopathic and homeopathic paradigms are incommensurable – both can not be correct and thus they can not really be considered complementary to each other.

Third, if it is the case that the patronage of CAM practitioners has dramatically increased in recent times, it is less than clear as to *why* this should be occurring. Again, it has not been the subject of much systematic research. Are 'push' or 'pull' factors more important to this development? Are patients voting with their feet towards CAM because they are dissatisfied with what conventional biomedicine has to offer; or are they particularly attracted by what CAM has to offer? One researcher who has examined this question is Siahpush (1999; see also Easthope 1993). Based upon multiple regression analysis of 787 Victorian telephone respondents, Siahpush found that the 'pull' of CAM was more significant than the 'push' from orthodox medicine.

In other work, Siahpush (1998) also evaluated why patronage of CAM is increasing. Again based upon detailed survey work in Australia, he concludes that the CAM social movement is mostly to be explained as the result of changing societal values towards what he calls postmodern values; a feature of which is a decline in the belief of the capacity of science and technology (in general, and medical science and technology in particular) to solve problems of modern life (see Bakx 1991).

Finally, any account of the rise of CAM would not be complete without mention of the backlash that has been generated from some sections of orthodox medicine. For instance, a journal has recently been established – *The Scientific Review of Alternative Medicine*. This journal will consider the evidence available for CAM by being 'devoted to the standard rational analysis of claims'. At the conference to launch this journal in the USA in early 1999, it was reported that

> speakers and most of the more than 200 delegates lambasted the growth of alternative medicine and the non-scientific theories behind them in an unabashedly one-sided assault. No-holds-barred attacks on alternative therapies were interspersed with critiques of the philosophical, political and psychological environment which surrounds their growing acceptance.

A former editor of a major medical journal was quoted as saying. 'There is no alternative medicine, there is only one medicine . . . which has been scientifically tested and works. Use it and pay for it' (quoted in *Medical Post* 1999).

Most tellingly perhaps, the editor of the newly launched journal was quoted as follows: 'Intellectually, most of the US and Canada do not accept the alternative medicine propaganda. I really believe (most people) think it's junk' (quoted in *Medical Post* 1999). Now assuming that he was quoted correctly (and if he then went on to support his belief with evidence the report didn't say), it is remarkable that he calls for evidence in one area yet apparently provided none for community acceptance, belief being sufficient. In other words, it appears that it is hoped by some that EBM will provide a stick with which to beat CAM, thus providing a new tool for orthodoxy in the ongoing historical struggle to undermine and marginalise CAM at one level while, at another, selectively co-opting and incorporating aspects of CAM treatment into orthodox practice.

The benefits of EBM for CAM

Having reviewed the emergence of both EBM on one hand and the apparent rise in demand for CAM services on the other, the impact of one on the other can now be considered. This question has been the subject of review in both the UK (Vincent and Furnham 1997) and US contexts (Spencer and Jacobs 1999). Here, it is argued that EBM has, and will progressively continue to have, both benefits and drawbacks for CAM.

The benefits are substantial and arise from the emphasis on outcomes rather than explanations. If a treatment works (to be shown to do more good than harm by rigorous Randomised Controlled Trial (RCT) methodology) then the explanation for its effectiveness is less important. If a treatment works and is safe, it deserves a place in the pantheon of accepted treatments and should be a part at least of a range of care options available to patients.

This feature of EBM is a big step forward for CAM. The finding that homeopathic treatment of hay fever works becomes far more important than explaining such therapeutic effect (see Reilly *et al.* 1986). Likewise, if using tiger balm for tension headaches is as effective as paracetamol and superior to a placebo (Schnatter and Randerson 1996), it is the outcome that is important not the underlying paradigm of disease causation or treatment. Basically, this approach means commensurability is less of an issue.

This represents a significant advance for CAM because, historically, it was the incommensurability (more usually expressed as incompatibility) of CAM modalities with conventional biomedicine that was the basis for the opposition and ridicule of unorthodox colleagues by organised medicine. A good example is chiropractic. In the Australian context, the long-standing hostility of the Australian Medical Association towards chiropractors was based upon an alleged incommensurability between orthodox medicine and the chiropractic theory of disease being caused by subluxations or veterbral misalignments (see Willis 1989). Yet various inquiries had questioned this view. In a perhaps visionary anticipation of EBM, the landmark New Zealand inquiry into chiropractic in the 1970s concluded that organised medicine's opposition to the theory of chiropractic (the theory of vertebral subluxation) was a 'red herring' (NZ Commission of Inquiry into Chiropractic 1979; also see Dew, Chapter 4). In other words, commensurability of paradigms is less important than outcomes. EBM has confirmed this development.

So what matters in EBM terms is not *why* CAM treatments work but *whether* they do. Evaluations of CAM treatments have begun to appear on EBM websites as the number of trials (of varying degrees of adequacy) of CAM treatments increases (for example, on the website Bandolier see http://www.jr2.ox.ac.uk:80/bandolier/band18/b18-3.html). In a sense, EBM provides a common ground on which both orthodox and unorthodox medicine can meet, in the form of the RCT-based methodology of EBM. In 2001 there were forty-four completed reviews of CAM treatments in the library of the Cochrane Collaboration (see http://www.rccm.org.uk/cochrane.htm) with another twenty-four protocols where reviews are in progress (see also Vickers 1999).

There are other social forces at work which are also promoting this rapprochement between orthodox and unorthodox healthcare. Most important is the growth of the consumer health movement, a central plank of which has been the plea 'Let's leave internecine struggle aside; if it helps patients and reduces the burden of sickness in the community, it doesn't matter who provides it; let's have it!' Thus, there is a trend towards consumers being less willing to accept the orthodox medical profession's hegemony over healthcare delivery and decision-making. Such a trend has been accelerated with the advent of the world wide web.

The combination of these social forces has resulted in a growth of interest in CAM. The evidence on increasing utilisation has led to several responses. For-profit health organisations and providers see a profit to be made and have begun to offer reimbursement. Universities in many parts of the world have established centres to research and explore the efficacy of hitherto 'alternative' treatments, most often under the title of 'integrative medicine'. Conferences are regularly held on topics such as the integration of CAM into conventional healthcare settings, including how CAM practitioners might operate in these settings.

The drawbacks of EBM for CAM

However, EBM is not all good news for CAM. It will be increasingly harder for CAM practitioners to sustain more esoteric treatments in the face of patient and community calls for evidence of effectiveness. There are also additional drawbacks and the following are some of the major issues that appear important.

The first relates to the emergent nomenclature of integrative medicine. Any understanding of the history of medical treatments leads us to view such emerging nomenclature with some reservations (Willis 1989). If it means integrating orthodox and unorthodox medical treatments so as to maximise the benefit to the patient, that is a benefit to all concerned and one that few would disagree with. But integration to a sceptical sociological gaze may also mean 'takeover'. There are plenty of instances where previously unorthodox healing practices were incorporated into orthodox medicine and the original practitioners shut out. Anaesthesiology is one example (see Krause 1997); X-rays are another (see Daly and Willis 1989). The dangers for CAM are obvious. Orthodox medicine will take over those CAM treatments that are found to be effective according to EBM methodology and then will argue that only those with medical training should administer them. Examples abound but two might be mentioned here. One is acupuncture: in the Australian context it was strenuously argued before an official government inquiry that the practice of acupuncture should be restricted to practitioners qualified in orthodox medicine (O'Neill 1994). The amount of training in acupuncture most orthodox medical practitioners had received was equated by non-medically qualified ('lay') acupuncturists at the inquiry as akin to a first aid course. The other example is chiropractic where there has long existed a view that the most suitable strategy for dealing with chiropractic was for orthodox medical practitioners (or at least their physical/physiotherapists colleagues) to start performing manipulation themselves.

The second set of factors relates to what might be called the politics of trials. Every inquiry ever held into CAM has called for more RCTs to be performed. It has proved difficult to adjudge the appropriate place of CAM in the heath services of a nation when evidence of effectiveness or otherwise is unavailable. In some cases there have even been recommendations that a specific sum of money be set aside to permit these to be performed. Yet relatively few RCTs of CAM have been performed. They are expensive and, in an era of withdrawal of state funding which has impacted particularly upon biomedical research, governments have been reluctant to fund such research on CAM. What trials there have been are often difficult to locate, possibly due to a 'publication bias' on the part of conventional medical journals.

An example of this is given in a study by Knipschild (1993) who searched for RCTs on the effectiveness of homeopathy. He found a substantial 'grey' or 'fugitive' literature. A search of Medline/Embase (until 1991) revealed eighteen published reports of controlled trials on homeopathy. Working through the bibliographies of these revealed twenty-eight more. Knipschild then embarked on a detailed search for the fugitive literature which turned up more than double this amount: more than 100 controlled studies. 'Our subsequent meta-analysis showed, to our astonishment, beneficial effects for homeopathy in many (but not all) well designed studies' (Knipschild 1993: 1136).

Most RCTs continue to be funded by drug companies in order to meet the legislative requirements for registration of new pharmaceutical substances. The result has been, in effect, to discourage research into non-pharmaceutical treatments for common complaints (hypertension and symptoms of menopause being two examples). In addition, most (but by no means all) CAM treatments have been for more minor ailments and not life-threatening conditions. However chronic and debilitating these may be, in a situation of scarcity, research into these ailments has, perhaps understandably, been accorded a lower priority.

There are also difficulties with the application of RCT methodology to CAM. Part of the RCT methodology involves holding constant as many variables as possible to control for, and allowing measurement of, their effect. RCT methodology works best where the treatment is quite straightforward. CAM treatments most often involve a combination of treatments tailored to individual patients, making the RCT methodology difficult to follow. Simplifying and narrowing the CAM treatment to enable an RCT to be devised may reduce the likely therapeutic effect of the treatment in the first place.

In addition there are issues about implementation and compliance. The danger is of a double standard when many areas of orthodox medicine have not been evaluated (see Imrie and Ramsey 2000). Already it has been observed in a number of areas of orthodox medicine that findings from a rigorous EBM process of evaluation have not been implemented in practice. An example is the drug Zantac (see Warren and Marshall 1983; Collyer 1996). In spite of the demonstration that stomach ulcers are the result of the bacteria *heliobacter pylori* and therefore susceptible to treatment with antibiotics, high levels of prescription of the drug Zantac continue. In other words, the impact of EBM is being weakened by a failure to act on the findings and to implement them in actual medical practice. Compliance it seems, is not only a problem amongst patients. If it is an issue for orthodox medicine, it is likely to be even more so for CAM. Appropriately applied EBM methodology has the potential to be as devastating for 'accepted wisdom' in CAM treatments as it is for conventional medicine.

The third set of factors relates to how EBM methodology is being used at the level of health funding and health policy. Already there is some disquiet about this effect within orthodox medicine, with concerns about EBM being a tool for cost-cutting and managerial co-optation involving a threat to professionals' clinical autonomy (see McDonald and Daly 2000; McLaughlin 2001). Sackett *et al.* (1997: 5) have responded to this claim by arguing that EBM will not necessarily reduce costs. As he puts it, 'Doctors practising evidence-based medicine will identify and apply the most efficacious interventions to maximise the quality and quantity of life for individual patients; this may raise rather than lower the cost of their care.' However, as one reviewer has argued, 'Dare I suggest that there will always be far greater eagerness to stop what is unproven rather than there will be to provide true extra funding for EBM-supported new services' (Sharp 1996: 1297). Furthermore, orthodox medical practitioners using CAM modalities are also caught up in this process, revealing the complexity of the issues involved. In one English study of GPs practising CAM, these medicines were found to be a useful resource with which some attempted to defend their clinical autonomy from what they perceived to be the threat of EBM (Adams 2000).

If this is a danger with EBM for orthodox medicine, it is even more of a threat for CAM. If only those therapeutic interventions for which evidence of their effectivness exists are to be supported, what to do about those interventions where there have been no trials to speak of and no acceptable (level I or II type) evidence to be able to draw conclusions one way or the other? Such is the case for the bulk of CAM treatments. It is one thing to only fund those interventions which have evidence; it is quite another, and a very political use of EBM, to decline to fund or support those interventions on which there is no acceptable evidence.

Legitimacy questions

So EBM is a mixed bag for CAM: advantageous in parts, less so in others. What will be its relation to and its impact upon the advancement of

CAM? Our argument is that these questions are determined by other social processes of which EBM type issues are likely to be only one part. Utilising the sociological concept of legitimation facilitates an understanding of these social processes.

The concept of legitimation, developed originally by the founding sociologist Max Weber, has been refined by the Frankfurt School critical theorist, Habermas (1970, 1976). It refers to the process whereby a set of practices is accepted as authoritative and becomes hegemonic. One of us has found it useful in the past in analysing CAM to distinguish between different types of legitimacy: clinical, scientific and politico-legal (see Willis 1989). Politico-legal legitimacy refers to acceptance in the wider society in general and the health system in particular. A healing modality may be said to have politico-legal legitimacy when its occupational territory is legislatively protected by statutory registration, its fees are refunded by various payment organisations including national state-funded health insurance schemes (where these exist), its practitioners are trained within the state-supported higher education system, and so on. There are two possible bases for politico-legal legitimacy: scientific on the one hand and clinical on the other. EBM is clearly a refinement of the grounds for scientific legitimacy; the extent to which the theories and treatments used by the modality in its healing practices can be supported by evidence according to the standards of science. Clinical legitimacy, on the other hand, refers to continuing patronage of practitioners by consumers willing to pay for their services.

Analysis of the history of health services shows that, as a basis for politico-legal legitimacy, clinical legitimacy is more important than scientific legitimacy (Willis 1989). We can take chiropractic as an example. This modality survived and now thrives to the point of substantial politico-legal legitimacy (even in the face of medical hostility), not because of scientifically acceptable evidence but because of ongoing clinical legitimacy: patients kept returning in large enough numbers because they received relief from musculo-skeletal related health problems.

What is the likely impact of EBM in the present and the future on the process of legitimacy? Our guess is minimal impact. Social processes external to the health system predominate. As evidence, two current examples from the EBM era in Australia are cited.

Traditional Chinese medicine (TCM)

Practitioners of TCM in Australia have long sought politico-legal legitimacy. In 1997, the state of Victoria commissioned a study to review the scientific evidence relating to TCM (in which one of us, Willis, had minor first-hand involvement) (Victorian Government Department of Human Services 1997). The interest of the then conservative Victorian government was public safety as there had previously been a small number of deaths from the inappropriate administration of TCM treatments. It seemed that, in the wrong hands, TCM treatments might not be as harmless as had previously been thought. The study team commissioned a respected senior clinician and health services researcher to evaluate all the evidence, that is, RCTs and other evidence that could be located in a wide search of the literature, including that in both Chinese and English language. The best that could be concluded from this review was that the evidence for the effectiveness of TCM is patchy: some exists but there are many areas that have simply never been studied using EBM-type methodology.

However, this finding of the patchy scientific legitimacy for TCM had little effect. The report was launched by the then Premier himself, and a subsequent ministerial review of TCM (of which Willis was also a member) was initiated. In spite of the general societal trend towards deregulation of labour markets being pursued as part of economic rationalist type policies (especially in the blue-collar arena), a recommendation for statutory registration was made and legislation eventually passed by the incoming state Government in the year 2000. Under this act, The Chinese Medicine Registration Board of Victoria was appointed by the Victorian Minister of Health, and has set about implementing a registration system for Chinese medicine practitioners (see http://www.cmrb.vic.gov.au/). Other Australian states have indicated a willingness and intention to implement mirror legislation. So, in this substantial politico-legal advance, scientific legitimacy in the form of solid EBM-type findings was not important.

Natural therapies

Another example is that of natural therapists. A huge boost in politico-legal legitimacy has recently been gained as a by-product of wider political changes in Australian society as a whole.

In the federal election in Australia in 1998, the third party of Australian politics, the Australian Democrats, gained the balance of power in the Senate, the Upper House of the Australian parliament. In order to secure passage of its taxation legislation introducing a Good and Services Tax into Australia, the Democrats and the conservative government of the day arrived at a political compromise. Part of the agreed package had a huge advantage for natural therapists (*The Age* 1999).

The minor advantage was a three-year exemption from the Goods and Services Tax (GST). The major advantage, however, was a promise to pursue a cohesive national accreditation system for naturopaths, herbalists and acupuncturists. This has been the aim of naturopathic organisations for more than a decade. In February 2002, the Australian Commonwealth government funded a project entitled 'Complementary Therapies Funding Program for the Establishment of Uniform Registration Systems for Suitably Qualified Practitioners in Acupuncture, Herbal Medicine and Naturopathy'.

It was designed to assist professional associations to devise such a registration system, especially around entrance standards, so that the GST-free status could be continued past the three-year limit (see Khoury 2002). The important point here is that EBM was nowhere to be seen. Even the most ardent naturopathic practitioner or patient would have to admit that there is relatively little scientific evidence of an EBM nature available to support such an advancement. Instead, its basis is clinical legitimacy; the plank to support the natural therapies has been a part of Australian Democrat policies since its inception as they sought to appeal to a particular constituency. The particular historical conjuncture gave the political opportunity to implement such a policy.

Conclusion

This chapter relates two important social movements currently affecting healthcare: EBM and CAM. The effect of EBM on CAM is, and will be, mixed. From the point of view of CAM practitioners there will be advantages and disadvantages. But caution should be exercised in expecting EBM to significantly influence the important question about the legitimacy, and appropriate role, of CAM therapies in the health services of the nation. Such questions are more likely to be resolved by social processes external to the health system itself.

Nonetheless, we do not suggest that the pursuit of EBM research on the effectiveness of CAM is not worthwhile. Such an approach could and should help resolve many of the day-to-day health policy funding questions. For this reason, it seems that the time may be appropriate for the establishment of institutions, perhaps modelled along the lines of the National Institutes of Health based National Centre for Complementary and Alternative Medicine in the USA, with a specifically garnered budgetary allocation to allow research (both RCT and other). The Bethesda, Maryland-based organisation, according to its mission statement 'conducts and supports basic and applied research and training and disseminates information on complementary and alternative medicine to practitioners and the public' (see http://nccam.nih.gov).

While EBM is a mixed blessing for CAM, CAM practitioners also cannot afford to stand outside these developments. Instead, the challenge facing all health treatments (orthodox as well as CAM) is to 'put its research efforts where its mouth is': that is, embrace the task of demonstrating effectiveness. If RCTs are at the heart of EBM as the 'gold standard' for evaluating effectiveness, then a Chinese proverb, cited by Eisenberg (quoted in Yamey 2000), is also worth remembering: 'Real gold does not fear even the hottest fire'. While EBM is not the beginning or the end of acting on this challenge, for CAM, climbing aboard is vital for future politico-legal legitimacy.

References

Adams, J. (2000) 'General Practitioners, complementary therapies and evidence-based medicine: the defence of clinical autonomy', *Complementary Therapies in Medicine* 8: 248–52.

Astin, J. (1998) 'Why patients use alternative medicine: results of a national study', *JAMA* 27,9(19): 1548–53.

Bakx, K. (1991) 'The "eclipse" of folk medicine in Western society', *Sociology of Health and Illness* 13: 20–39.

Berliner, H. and Salmon, J. (1980) 'The holistic alternative to scientific medicine: history and analysis', *International Journal of Health Services* 10,1: 133–14.

Collyer, F. (1996) 'Understanding ulcers: medical knowledge, social constructionism and helicobacter pylori', *Annual Review of Health Social Sciences* 6: 1–41.

Daly, J. (forthcoming) *Mining for Gold: the search for a science of clinical care,* San Francisco: University of California Press.

Daly, J. and Willis, E. (1989) 'Technological innovation and the labour process in health care', *Social Science & Medicine* 28,11: 1149–53.

Easthope, G. (1993) 'The response of orthodox medicine to the challenge of alternative medicine in Australia', *Australia and New Zealand Journal of Sociology* 29: 289–301

Eisenberg, D.M., Kessler, R.C. and Foster, C. *et al.* (1993) 'Unconventional medicine in the United states: prevalence, costs, and patterns of use', *New England Journal of Medicine* 328: 246–352.

Fisher, M. (ed.) (1989) *US Preventive Services Task Force. Guide to clinical preventive services: an assessment of the effectiveness of 169 interventions,* Baltimore: Williams and Wilkins.

Guyatt, G. (1993) 'Letter to the editor', *Journal of the American Medical Association* 269,10: 1255.

Habermas, J. (1970) 'Technology and science as ideology', in *Toward a Rational Society,* Boston: Beacon Press, pp. 81–122.

Habermas, J. (1976) *Legitimation Crisis,* London: Heinneman.

Imrie, R. and Ramsey, D. (2000) 'The evidence for evidence-based medicine', *Complementary Therapies in Medicine* 8: 123–6.

Kastner, M. and Burroughs, H. (1996) *Alternative Healing: the complete A–Z guide to more than 150 alternative therapies,* New York: Holt.

Kaufman, M. (1971) *Homeopathy in America: the rise and fall of a medical heresy,* Baltimore: Johns Hopkins Press.

Khoury, R. (2002) 'Government grants $0.5 million for GST-Free Registration System', *Journal of Australian Traditional Medicine Society* 8,1: 7–8.

Knipschild, P. (1993) 'Searching for alternatives: loser pays', *Lancet* 341: 1136.

Krause, E. (1997) *Power and Illness,* New York: Elsevier.

Kuhn, T. (1962) *The Structure of Scientific Revolutions,* Chicago: University of Chicago Press.

MacLennan, A.H., Wilson, D.H. and Taylor, A.W. (1996) 'Prevalence and cost of alternative medicine in Australia', *Lancet* 347: 569–73.

McDonald, I. and Daly, J. (2000) 'The anatomy and relations of evidence-based medicine', *Australian and New Zealand Journal of Medicine* 30,3: 385–92.

McLaughlin, J. (2001) 'EBM and risk: rhetorical resources and the articulation of professional identity', *Journal of Management in Medicine* 15,5: 352–63.

Medical Post (1999) 'Science meets alternative medicine'. Online. Available HTTP: http://www.mdlink.com/mdlink/english/members/medpost/data/3511/17B.HTM 35,11: (16 March).

National Health and Medical Research Council (NHMRC) (1995) *Guidelines for the Development and Implementation of Clinical Practice Guidelines*, Quality of Care and Health Outcomes Committee, Canberra: Australian Government Publishing Service: 39.

Neissen, L., Grijseels, E. and Rutten, F. (2000) 'The evidence-approach in health policy and healthcare delivery', *Social Science and Medicine* 51: 859–69.

New Zealand Commission of Inquiry into Chiropractic (1979) *Chiropractic in New Zealand: report of the Commission of Inquiry*, Wellington, N.Z.: P.D. Hasselberg, Government Printer.

O'Neill, A. (1994) *Enemies Within & Without: educating chiropractors, osteopaths and traditional acupuncturists*, Bundoora, Victoria: La Trobe University Press.

Paramore, L.C. (1997) 'Use of alternative therapies: estimates from the 1994 Robert Wood Johnson Foundation national access to care survey', *Journal of Pain Symptom Management* 13: 83–9.

Rangachari, P. (1997) 'Evidence based medicine: old French wine with a new Canadian label', *Joournal of the Royal Society of Medicine* 20: 280–4.

Reilly, D., Taylor, M., McSharry, C. and Aitchison, T. (1986) 'Is homoeopathy a placebo response? Controlled trial of homoeopathic potency, with pollen in hay-fever as model', *Lancet* ii: 881–6.

Reilly, D., Morag, A., Beattie, N., Campbell, J., et al. (1994) 'Is evidence for homoeopathy reproducible?', *Lancet* 344(8937): 1601–6.

Sackett, D., Strauss, S., Rosenberg, W., Richardson, S., Gray, J. and Haynes, B. (1996) 'Evidence-based medicine; what it is and what it isn't', *British Medical Journal* 312: 71–2.

Sackett, D., Richardson, S., Rosenberg, W. and Haynes, B. (1997) *Evidence-based Medicine*, London: Churchill Livingstone.

Sackett, D. (2000) 'The sins of expertness and a proposal for redemption', *British Medical Journal* 230, 6 May: 1283.

Schattner, P. and Randerson, D. (1996) 'Tiger balm as a treatment of tension headache. A clinical trial in general practice', *Australian Family Physician* 25(2): 216–20.

Sharp, D. (1996) 'Evidence-based medicine' (book reviews), *Lancet*, 9 Nov., 347: 9037, 1297.

Siahpush, M. (1998) 'Postmodern values, dissatisfaction with conventional medicine and popularity of alternative therapies', *Journal of Sociology* 34: 58–70.

Siahpush, M. (1999) 'Why do people favour alternative medicine', *Australia and New Zealand Journal of Public Health* 23: 266–71, 29: 289–301.

Spencer, J. and Jacobs, J. (1999) *Complementary/Alternative medicine: an evidence-based approach*, St Louis: Mosby.

Vickers, A. (1999) 'Editorial: evidence based medicine and complementary medicine', *Evidence based Medicine.* Online. Available HTTP: http://www.acpjc.org/Content/130/2/ISSUE/ACPJC-1999-130-2-A13.htm   (Nov–Dec: 168–9).

Victorian Government Department of Human Services (1997) *Review of Traditional Chinese Medicine,* Melbourne: Victorian Government printer. Online. Available HTTP: http://www.dhs.vic.gov.au/phd/hce/chinese/discpap/

Vincent, C. and Furnham, A. (1997) *Complementary Medicine,* Chichester: Wiley.

Warren, J. and Marshall, B. (1983) 'Unidentified curved bacilli on gastric epithelium in active chronic gastritis', *Lancet,* 1: 1283.

Willis, E. (1989) *Medical Dominance* (rev. edn), Sydney: Allen & Unwin.

Willis, E. and White, K. (forthcoming) 'Evidence based medicine, the medical profession and health policy', in Lin, V. and Gibson, B. (eds) *Competing Rationalities: evidence-based health policy,* Melbourne: Oxford University Press.

Yamey, G. (2000) 'Editorial: can complementary medicine be evidence-based?, *Western Journal of Medicine.* Online. Available HTTP: http://www.studentbmj.com/back_issues/1000/editorials/351.html (173: 4–5).

Chapter 4

The regulation of practice

Practitioners and their interactions
with organisations

Kevin Dew

Introduction

This chapter argues that all healing practices, including complementary and alternative medicine (CAM), are increasingly influenced by forms of regulation that progressively lead to their standardisation. The type of regulation varies over time and has different consequences. The relationship between regulation and notions of science is critical to the process of standardisation of practices, but it is not a straightforward one. The state, consumers or patients, the medical profession and its competitors have an interest in regulation. There are great tensions between these stakeholders, and how these tensions are resolved impacts upon the clinical freedom of practitioners and the choices available to those seeking therapeutic assistance. In the following, a brief outline of the history of the regulation of medicine is provided, and the trends in this regulation and its effects on both established medicine and CAM are explored. Regulatory trends are illustrated with reference to salient events in New Zealand.

Regulation, politics and education

The 1858 Medical Act in Britain was the culmination of a long, bitter and, on occasion, violent campaign by general practitioners to achieve statutory regulation (Waddington 1977). The Act set the standard for the regulation of medical practitioners in Britain and its colonies. It gave the General Medical Council (GMC) powers to control who could practice medicine by establishing a system of medical registration. Although not restricting the practice of medicine to doctors, the GMC was so powerful that it could veto other occupations' claims for recognition (Larkin 1983). Since this time, healthcare occupations such as nurses and physiotherapists have had to seek medical patronage in the same ways as the medical profession had previously sought state patronage (Larkin 1983).

The 1858 Act in Britain was not, however, an outright victory for the regular medical practitioners of the day. The popularity of homeopathy posed a serious challenge to orthodox medicine, and a clause was inserted into legislation that would ensure homeopaths could practise. Homeopathy has therefore been able to maintain a place in regulated medical practice in Britain – though a rather vulnerable place. Homeopathic physicians are licensed to practice under the National Health Service, and there were still five homeopathic hospitals operating within the NHS in 2001.

Apart from the homeopaths, the 1858 Medical Act had a dramatic impact in excluding alternative therapies. It took another 135 years before alternative therapies were able to gain recognition and favourable legislation as separate occupational groups. This occurred with the passing of the Osteopaths Act 1993 in the United Kingdom (Fisher and Ward 1994).

After the 1858 Act, Britain's colonies followed suit in regulating the medical profession. Legislation granting the medical profession advantages over its competitors occurred in Victoria, Australia, in 1862. By 1867, the first Act securing dominance and autonomy for the medical profession in New Zealand was passed. The 1867 Medical Practitioners Act incorporated a provision clearly aimed at undermining the strength of homeopathy in New Zealand. This provision was for the adoption of British pharmacopoeia as the only prescription source in public hospitals, leaving homeopathy out of the hospital system (Belgrave 1985).

But the New Zealand medical profession's new powers were quickly relinquished. In one province the government appointed a homeopath as an assessor to examine individuals' qualifications when applying to register as medical practitioners. In response to this, and the refusal of the government to cancel the appointment, members of the Medical Board resigned. The reaction to this by the government was the 1869 Act, which took the power to regulate medical practitioners away from the medical profession, and placed it in the hands of the Registrar-General (Belgrave 1985). It was not until 1914 that doctors would regain what they had lost in the 1869 legislation.

Though politicians were wary of granting doctors professional control of medicine in New Zealand, they continued to pass legislation which gave doctors more social and judicial powers. Doctors were given the role of providing scientific legitimacy to a series of legislative policies, including disease prevention, the supervision of private hospitals and the control of food and drug legislation. The position of medicine improved as the state made attempts to control the lives and activities of women. Contagious Diseases Acts were passed in the 1860s, which treated women suspected of prostitution as being morally corrupt and medically unclean (Wilson 1992). The 1869 Contagious Diseases Act gave doctors the powers to enforce the hospitalisation of prostitutes diagnosed with venereal disease, and also the right to medically inspect women suspected of being prostitutes (Belgrave 1985). The moral campaigns of the state increased the professional power of medicine.

The early state regulation of the medical profession did not depend upon any concern for therapeutic effectiveness, and was not based on scientific validation but related to the state's need to regulate the population and to effective lobbying by practitioners. There was an uneasy 'trust' between the state and the medical profession. However, with protective legislation the medical profession could exclude other healing occupations from accessing state benefits. As such, alternative medical worldviews had limited purchase in the public arena.

The socialisation of medical practitioners through their medical training extended the limitation of acceptable medical worldviews. Through the education and training of practitioners, regulation of practices is enforced – at least for the time of the training. A significant event in the relationship between science, medicine and regulation was the Flexner Report in North America (as mentioned by Turner in his Foreword to this volume).

In the early twentieth century, the American Medical Association invited the Carnegie Foundation to conduct an investigation of the 160 or so medical colleges in the USA and Canada. The resulting report, published in 1910 and known as the Flexner Report, objected to the lack of medical science in the curriculum. Abraham Flexner, the author, had an overtly mechanistic notion of health, referring to the body as 'an infinitely complex machine' and saw medicine as 'part and parcel of modern science' (Osheron and Amarasingham 1981: 228). The Report recommended that the great majority of schools should be closed and the 'first-rate' schools should be strengthened. After the Flexner Report the state examining boards barred graduates from schools with a low rating, regardless of the candidate's own knowledge or proficiency (Coulter 1973). The criterion used for the rating of schools was heavily weighted against the homeopathic schools. Schools which devoted more attention to pharmacology were downgraded, those with more pathological and chemical laboratories were favoured (Coulter 1973), and the Report recommended against the allocation of funds to homeopathic schools. The Report's recommendations were supported by philanthropic foundations, with financial support for scientific medicine coming from the Rockefeller and Carnegie foundations in the wake of the Report (Berliner 1984; Salmon 1984).

The New Zealand educational situation was very different from that of the USA. The first medical school was established in Otago in 1874, with only one other established since. The Otago Medical School was criticised for not being able to offer its students as much clinical experience as the better overseas schools, due to the small size of the teaching hospital in Dunedin. This criticism prompted the Otago School to offer a very conservative medical education to avoid further censure. Any educational experiences that were outside a strict orthodoxy might attract further concern about the educational standards of the Otago Medical School and therefore did not find their way on to the medical curriculum.

It can be noted here that New Zealand and Australia have very conformist medical establishments. England has the existence of homeopathic hospitals, and in the USA there have been successes for homeopathy, eclecticism and osteopathy, all having had periods of strength within the medical profession. A similar situation applies in Canada. By contrast, New Zealand trained doctors had no alternative educational experiences that would lead them to question 'scientific medicine' (Belgrave 1985).

Medical science and standardisation

It was not until well into the twentieth century that stronger links were made between science and medicine in relation to the regulation of practices. Here, science of a specific sort took on a central and powerful role in standardising therapies.

The occupation of medicine became professionalised during the age of heroic medicine, and gained state privileges as well as the exclusion of alternative therapies from such special consideration at this time. The age of heroic medicine dominated Europe and its colonies and the USA in the eighteenth and nineteenth centuries. Medical treatment during this period included bloodletting, administration of large doses of calomel (mercurous chloride) and other dangerous mineral drugs, purgatives, emetics and venesection (Kaufman 1971; Duffy 1979).

Benjamin Rush, a very influential exponent of this style of heroic medicine ascribed all disease to capillary tension and the only cure for this was bloodletting and purging (Duffy 1979). Rush believed that one of the hindrances to the development of medicine was the reliance on the powers of nature to cure disease (Duffy 1979). For Rush, desperate diseases required desperate remedies: 'He had such confidence in the lancet that he was willing to remove up to four-fifths of the blood in the body if necessary to alleviate the symptoms' (Kaufman 1971: 2).

General bloodletting was carried out by venesection, and local bloodletting by the use of leeches. Blistering was also a treatment of choice, where a second-degree burn would be created and would become infected and suppurate. The pus was seen as a sign of the infection being drawn out of the system (Kaufman 1971). Purging was carried out by the use of emetics to induce vomiting, and cathartics, to evacuate the bowels. Calomel was also given in large doses for a variety of conditions. These massive doses produced salivation, loosening of the teeth, falling out of the hair and other symptoms of acute mercury poisoning. For the patient, these reactions to the poisons were clear signs that the body was ridding itself of disease (Kaufman 1971; Rosenberg 1992).

Surgery was as perilous. The patient receiving surgery was likely to be drunk in order to numb the pain. The surgeon's hands and instruments were not sterile, and he was likely to have a frockcoat 'stiff with dried blood of previous patients, the whole atmosphere fraught with pain and thick with bacteria' (Sigsworth 1972: 109). Although Sigsworth suggests that this picture of surgery in the nineteenth century may be overstated, the surgical mortality rate was as high as 17 per cent in some hospitals (Sigsworth 1972).

From the perspective of contemporary medical beliefs it is difficult to understand why such drastic treatments were used and why they were not put to a test of effectiveness. In the nineteenth century the idea that statistical methods should be employed to decide if the differences in rates of cure between two populations of patients could be attributed to treatment was resisted by physicians (Porter 1995). It was not until the twentieth century that the peculiar medical research 'style of reasoning' (Hacking 1990) that is so familiar to us today developed. In terms of contemporary standards, any drugs used by medical practitioners in the nineteenth century were not standardised. Therefore, practitioners could only estimate the potency of the drugs they were giving. In 1910 the idea of the 'biological assay' was first mooted. At this time it was suggested that the biological potency of digitalis (from the leaves of the foxglove) could be assessed by a 'cat unit'. That is, pharmacists making up the potion could test the potency of the leaves by finding out how many leaves it took to kill a cat (Porter 1995). This solution to finding the strength of medicinal preparations was only very partial, as different cats varied in their tolerance for drugs. But from then on more effort was put into standardising medicines, and it was not until medicines themselves were standardised that one could put any faith in tests of therapeutic effectiveness.

In addition, to accept the notion of a controlled trial would be to subordinate clinical judgements and medical ideas to the dominance of numbers. Although attempts were made in the first half of the nineteenth century to assess the outcomes of some treatments by subjecting them to statistical tests, this was rejected as medicine was 'always concerned with the individual' and not with 'facts without authenticity' (Hacking 1990: 85). The use of statistical methods in medicine only began after 1900, and it was not until the 1940s that statistical tests gained a firm foothold in medical research.

One important concept that needed to be accepted before clinical trials could become the standard was the notion of the 'normal' that could be compared with the deviant (Hacking 1990). Without a notion of a normal distribution of the population it was not possible to establish whether the responses one got from a therapeutic intervention were due to chance (therefore not outside the normal distribution) or due to some real effect. The notion of normal that we use today, which is both a comparison with the pathological and an ideal that we strive for, did not take a hold on medical and social thought until the late nineteenth century.

In medicine the notion of normality and standardising found its apotheosis in the randomised controlled trial (RCT). Evidence-based medicine (EBM) as currently used places RCTs at the top of the hierarchy of authoritative evidence (see Willis and White, Chapter 3). A RCT in medicine is where a treatment is given to one group of people (the experimental group) and not another (the control group). People are allocated to the groups on a random basis. However, in order to see whether a treatment is better than placebo, neither the control group nor the experimental group must know whether they are being given the treatment. The treatment and the non-treatment must appear the same to everyone. In a further complication it is ideal if RCTs are also 'double blind': that is, neither the patient nor the person giving the treatment should know whether the treatment is the real one or a fake one. If the person giving the agent knows it is the treatment and not the fake, they can produce a 'healing' effect or placebo effect that is not related to the agent under study.

This means that RCTs are particularly appropriate for certain types of treatment. It is easy to test a drug, as you can design a placebo to look exactly like the treatment. It is very difficult (if not impossible) to submit surgery, counselling, spinal manipulation and many other forms of treatment to a true double blind RCT, although non-double blind RCTs may still be possible. RCTs are also based on certain assumptions about disease and healing. One is that all people are essentially the same. If you have a disease then you will react in essentially the same way as I will, and we will also both react to a treatment for that disease in the same way. In other words, treatments and people can be treated homogeneously. But some healing systems start from a different assumption – that we are all unique, and that even if you and I have the same disease, you will react differently from me and we will respond to different therapeutic approaches (Dew 2001). If we hold the latter assumption, RCTs have very limited value. Because of the different assumptions that people make about health and the human response to illness, we have no universal agreement on what constitutes evidence. We have a dominant view, which over time changes.

However, once established as ideals, RCTs could be used rhetorically to criticise and limit the practices of other therapeutic systems. The standardised procedures of science and their dominance are illustrated by the case of the Commission of Inquiry into Chiropractic (CIC) in New Zealand. This is in some ways paradoxical, as the chiropractors won a major victory over the medical profession, but that victory came at the cost of subordination to scientific medicine. This case indicates the complex processes of intertwining politics and science in the regulation of therapeutic practices.

The politics and science of chiropractic

There are a host of interesting issues that came out of the New Zealand CIC, and these have been discussed elsewhere (Dew 1998, 2000). The focus here is on the disputes over science and the process of limitation of practice. Prior to the extensive CIC in 1978/9, limited support had been given to chiropractic and osteopathy in Australia from other inquiries – the *Ward Report* in 1975 and the *Webb Report* in 1977. These reports recommended that chiropractors and osteopaths be restricted to neuro-musculoskeletal disorders rather than being able to treat a range of organic or visceral disorders (Willis 1983: 186).

Not surprisingly, a lack of scientific support to validate chiropractic was a very common theme in the submissions to the CIC that opposed chiropractic. By contrast, the chiropractors appealed to popular support to validate their claims. This supports Willis's view that the medical profession demand scientific legitimacy for chiropractic, whilst chiropractors offered clinical legitimacy (Willis 1983). Political support and lobbying led to successful legislation for the medical profession in the nineteenth century, but in the twentieth century the medical profession attempted to deny this avenue to the chiropractors, citing 'science' as the route to legitimacy.

According to a New Zealand Medical Association (NZMA) submission, patients benefited from chiropractic due to a sharing of faith in manipulation and spontaneous remission of the condition. The only way of eliminating these effects was through a RCT. In a Health Department submission, John McKinlay, Professor of Sociology at Boston University, argued that effectiveness must be proven before a treatment was publicly funded. One issue he had to contend with related to the flood of letters (13,000 in all) that the CIC received from chiropractic patients. McKinlay argued that submissions from patients were worthless in assessing effectiveness because they were opinion (CIC transcript: 448). Medical submissions attacked the way in which chiropractors used this public support: 'Neither the government nor the medical profession decides by a vote which therapy is scientifically valid. Such a determination is made by the researcher and clinicians employing the technology of modern scientific discovery' (written submission made by Dr Katz to the CIC 1979: 58).

Related to the 'effectiveness' debate was one on the scope of chiropractic treatment. The NZMA argued that chiropractors considered it within their rightful province to treat a diverse range of conditions: 'It is inconceivable [to us] that hypertension, whooping-cough and diabetes, as claimed, are in any way due to spinal malalignment; and culpable to suggest that they be treated by chiropractic adjustment' (opening written submission made by the NZMA to the CIC 1979: 13).

The NZMA submissions went on to suggest that chiropractic 'was founded as an *alternative* system of medicine in opposition to orthodox practice, and remains so in doctrine' (Boyd-Wilson 1978: 17). By contrast, the chiropractors gave a definition of chiropractic to demonstrate that it had made changes from the original claims of its founders that many diseases are caused by spinal misalignment:

> Chiropractic is that science and art which utilizes the inherent recupera-tive powers of the body and deals with the relationship between the nervous system and the spinal column, including the immediate articu-lations and the role of this relationship in the restoration and mainte-nance of health.
> (Opening written submission made by the NZCA to the CIC 1979: 23)

In this definition, chiropractors avoided making claims about treating any particular condition, such as whooping cough, but offered a general approach to all conditions. The chiropractors went further in accepting the ground of the debate as laid down by the medical profession. Chiropractors themselves argued that the clinical evidence on spinal manipulation influen-cing internal organ function, the most controversial claim of chiropractors and osteopaths, 'is sketchy and based primarily on anecdotal reporting and opinion originating from individual experience together with the occasional uncontrolled trial' and that the link was only a possibility (written sub-mission made by Dr Haldeman to the CIC 1979: 29).

The CIC were persuaded by this attempt to position chiropractic within a framework acceptable to medicine. The 'sketchy' nature of the evidence about influence on internal organs, and its anecdotal nature, are exactly the criticisms that the medical profession levelled at chiropractic in general. The abandonment of what some might have seen as the central tenets of chiropractic philosophy became an important feature in the gaining of credibility for that profession. The 'scientific' evidence was as debatable in the case of chiropractic improving back pain as it was in chiropractic improving asthma, but the medical profession would not brook, under any circumstances, the possibility of the latter. This situated chiropractic as a speciality rather than as an alternative healing system. Yet, at the same time, the chiropractors did not want to place limits around what this speciality could do. They argued that 'Chiropractors do not contend that subluxation, however defined, is the most significant causal factor in disease' but suggested that 'in the current state of knowledge it is both unscientific and meaningless to endeavour to limit the range of conditions amenable to Chiropractic therapy' (closing written submission made by the NZCA to the CIC 1979: 19).

The CIC found in support of the chiropractors, and was very critical of the medical profession. The CIC recommended that chiropractors gain access to state health benefits that were available to medical doctors for the treatment of back problems and was critical of medical practitioners using manual therapy. It argued that 'what evidence we have received is largely that of patients whose experience of attempts at manual therapy by their own doctor drove them to a chiropractor' (CIC 1979: 31). Due to the specialised nature of spinal manual therapy it was recommended that chiropractors should be responsible for training. Chiropractors should also have access to hospitals (CIC 1979: 5). The CIC dismissed the arguments made by McKinlay and instead found 'as a fact that chiropractic treatment aimed at the relief of musculo-skeletal symptoms does demonstrate an ability to provide such relief' (CIC 1979: 285). This 'fact' was not discovered on the basis of clinical trials, as McKinlay would have it.

The recommendations of the Inquiry were however diluted with the process of implementation, a process that could be seen as eliminating the possibility of chiropractic seriously challenging orthodox medicine in New Zealand. Chiropractors did not secure access to hospitals or take over training in spinal manipulation for other health professionals.

Despite the overwhelming support of chiropractic, the Commission was not prepared to give chiropractors the prestige and privilege of the medical profession. In a very insightful passage the Commission claimed that:

> If chiropractors had limited their practices solely to cases of backache, and if some of them had not gone beyond the limits of reasonable professional conduct, it is unlikely that they would have antagonised the organised medical profession to the degree that became evident as the Commission's hearings proceeded. In fact, some chiropractors claim that their treatment is capable of relieving a great variety of conditions apart from backache: asthma, deafness, diabetes, high blood pressure, and bed wetting are only a few examples of the wide range of disorders for which chiropractic is claimed to be of at least potential benefit.
>
> (CIC 1979: 27)

The CIC denied chiropractic the position of being an alternative form of therapy. Instead, chiropractic is positioned as offering services complementary to the medical profession. The CIC concluded that 'chiropractors do not provide an alternative comprehensive system of healthcare, and should not hold themselves out as doing so' and those who did should be subjected to 'drastic disciplinary action' (CIC 1979: 4).

Following the release of the *Report* by the CIC, the NZMA moved to support the initiation of a clinical trial to compare medical management, physiotherapy and chiropractic manipulation for back and neck pain (*NZMJ* 1980a). However, even though the medical profession was highly critical of chiropractors for not subjecting their claims to RCTs, when it came to their attempts to organise such a trial a host of obstacles appeared. Problems included: the large number of patients required; the inability to deal with 'important' questions in the treatment of back pain, such as the psychological and postural factors involved; a lack of diagnostic specificity; the inability to make the trials double blind; the inability to standardise treatment; the ethical issue raised when using placebos meant the withholding of treatment; and the difficulty in assessing outcomes (*NZMJ* 1980b; Gow 1981). Chiropractic was criticised by medicine for producing no scientific evidence but, when it came to a comparative trial, the medical establishment itself claimed that such scientific evidence was too difficult to obtain.

A consequence of the Inquiry is that the limitation of chiropractic claims can be clearly seen. In order to become acceptable, the chiropractors had to pose no threat to the niche occupied by general practitioners. This limitation of chiropractic has been commented on by other authors in different countries. Saks (1994) argues that alternative practitioners frequently dilute the radicalism of their ideas, citing the example of the restricted claims for chiropractic made by the Anglo-European College of Chiropractic in Britain. Coburn notes a similar process in Canada where some provinces have given official recognition to chiropractic as a self-governing health occupation but at the expense of narrowing the scope of what can be practised. Coburn goes so far as to say that chiropractic has been tamed and medicalised (Coburn 1993a, 1993b). Similar arguments have been made about chiropractors in Australia (Clavarino and Yates 1995).

In conclusion, the regulation of chiropractic became dependent on categorising it as compatible with medicine. The therapeutic systems could not be allowed to compete. As such, the medically 'untenable' claims made by chiropractors had to be rejected. Chiropractic went from being a radical alternative without access to state funding, to an adjunct to medical practice with access to state funding. Chiropractic achieved this move not by scientific validation in the limited sense called for by the medical profession, but by popular support. However, this recognition was limited to the treatment of musculo-skeletal conditions. The notions of 'scientific medicine' were to dominate chiropractic, although the requirement to submit to scientific trials was not met. However, new forms of regulation have since developed that have the potential to further limit therapeutic practices.

Accountability and quality assurance

The development of EBM, with RCTs as the most authoritative evidence, provides a powerful form of standardising therapeutic practices (see Willis and White, Chapter 4). If a treatment does not meet the standards set by RCTs, then the treatment has an inferior status. The outcome of the CIC indicates how ideals can be undermined by politics and popular support. In addition, once in their own practice any practitioner can choose whatever therapy they like, RCT-validated or not, if there are no strong measures accounting for what they do. However, the eventual linkage between EBM and quality assurance further standardises and limits therapeutic practice.

The development of quality assurance (QA) in medicine (and its associated developments such as Continuous Quality Improvement, clinical governance, revalidation and recertification) links closely to science and education. QA puts in place mechanisms that allow tighter control over what practitioners can do. As a general definition, QA:

> refers to programmes that set standards, assess the performance of professionals or institutions with respect to these standards, encourage improvement where performance can be improved, and attempt corrective action where the non-compliance is unacceptable.
>
> (Jost 1992: 70)

Programmes include peer reviews of practitioners by colleagues or by external agents, individual practitioner medical audits, continuing medical education and other activities.

Prior to the 1980s there were no explicit references made to QA in healthcare, though systems for specifying, checking and maintaining quality had been developing since the 1960s in Britain and the USA because of the increasing costs of health services (Ellis and Whittington 1993). QA developments in England were the result of governmental concerns with efficiency, consumer service, businesslike management and accountability in the National Health Service, and the drive by Royal Colleges and others to improve the practice of medicine (Jost 1992). The British government confronted QA issues directly in a 1989 Health Service White Paper produced by the Department of Health, *Working for Patients*, which proposed that compulsory medical audit programmes be established in both the hospital and primary care sector (Seale 1993). The method of medical audit comes from the USA, where audits were imposed upon doctors by insurance companies in order to limit the cost of medical care (Seale 1993).

In both the USA and the UK medical audit is carried out through peer review, which means that senior doctors retain control over the process and regulate their juniors (Allsop and Mulcahy 1996; Curtis and Taket 1996). In the New Zealand case, we also see the concern that medical audit and other QA measures allow for the greater regulation of more marginalised groups within the medical profession.

The practice of doctors retaining control of the process is justified on the basis of the notion of clinical freedom – yet the process of standardisation through EBM appears, ironically, to contradict that notion. Arguments have been made that medical practice should be evidence based and firmly embedded in science (Berg 1997). Such developments have the potential to narrow the focus of medical practice and restrict the autonomy of the medical practitioner. This is of particular importance to medical practitioners who may practice some form of therapy that does not conform to currently accepted conventions of medical practice, and whose treatment cannot easily be submitted to the gold standard of medical research – the RCT. The link with QA is that developments in this field, such as peer review and medical audit, are likely to be increasingly based on EBM. With EBM there is a hierarchy of evidence, with RCTs being at the top, various forms of experimental design coming next, and consensus of experts following. All of these processes of determining evidence are based on the authority of the normal distribution, standard populations and standard treatment, or the authority of orthodoxy.

Developments in QA are linked to guidelines of 'good practice'. One of the ways in which ambiguity is reduced amidst medical uncertainty is by the development of protocols. Terms like guidelines, protocols and practice policies have been used to describe the same thing, which can be translated as 'a set of *instructions* telling medical personnel to do a certain thing in a certain situation' (Berg 1997: 52). Once protocols are established, failure to follow them is likely to be treated as a serious error in itself, regardless of patient outcome (Daniels 1992). This suggests that the development of a consensus is required to deal with the endemic uncertainty of medical practice, and the heretical doctor who threatens this consensus.

The relationship between QA and the standardisation of therapeutic practices is well illustrated by the Medical Practitioners Act 1995 (MPA) in New Zealand. The MPA 1995 is specifically related to medical doctors; however, it provides a blueprint for other health-related occupational groups attempting to gain more state regulation. In 2003 it is anticipated that a Health Professionals' Competency Assurance Act will be passed by the New Zealand Parliament. Much of this Act will be based on the MPA 1995, and many alternative practitioners will be regulated by the Act.

The MPA 1995 can be seen as a strategy of the medical profession to maintain professional control through putting in place mechanisms that ensure homogeneity amongst medical practitioners. This effort links with the state's concern to rationalise the delivery of medical services in order to control costs. That is, in both instances there is a drive towards standardisation of practices. For the state, this is to ensure comparability allowing for the possible identification of areas where cost savings can be made. For the medical profession, standardisation is one element in ensuring the credibility of the profession in the eyes of its funding agents and in the eyes of the public, particularly in times where the medical profession has come under much criticism. Ethical lapses amongst the medical profession and concerns over the cost of medical services and the possible waste of resources have acted to influence the development of QA in medicine.

The MPA 1995 incorporated a number of changes from the previous legislation that gave the medical disciplinary and professional bodies more extensive powers. The Medical Council already had an array of powers at its disposal to control its membership, including the ability to fine, impose working restrictions, and suspend or expel a practitioner. Since the passage of the MPA 1995, the Council gained the power to order an assessment of a practitioner, whether or not a complaint had been lodged against that practitioner, and also to implement or oversee QA and competency programmes for its members. The Medical Council was granted the power to impose a recertification programme upon a practitioner where they may be required to, among other things, pass an examination, have their clinical practices assessed, and do 'anything else that the Council considers appropriate' (Medical Practitioners Act 1995: 34). These powers give the Medical Council the potential to have greater control over the clinical practice of individual practitioners, and if they fail to meet any set national benchmark the Medical Council has the power to suspend a practitioner's registration or practising certificate.

During the hearings on the MPA 1995, representatives of the medical profession had to justify their increase in powers and their ability to further control their membership. One way to do this was to argue that medical practice was based on the 'gold standard' of RCTs. But this strategy was not sustainable, as the parliamentarians on the Committee were well aware that much of medical practice could not be so justified. However, the more flexible concept of EBM could be used to give the profession an image of being based on a sound foundation.

Although representatives of the medical profession may appeal to the need for greater public accountability to justify the development of EBM, this comes at the cost of consumer choice. This is exemplified in the debate over Clause 58/4 in the MPA 1995. In the original draft of the Act, this clause from the previous legislation had been dropped. Clause 58/4 stated that 'No person shall be guilty of disgraceful conduct in a professional respect merely because he has adopted and practised any theory of medicine or surgery, if in so doing he has acted honestly and in good faith' (Cole 1985: 541).

In a submission representing consumer interests, a chairperson of a community health group argued that the dropping of the clause allowing clinical freedom would force doctors to stop practising complementary therapies. The suggestion is that alternative medicine would not fit within the paradigm of EBM, as much of what is practised is not amenable to RCTs and is unlikely to be accepted by a consensus of experts. Similar concerns were expressed over the development of QA measures where practitioners would have to submit to peer review and medical audit. This was seen as a way of standardising practices and eliminating those who offered alternative views. In the end, the Medical Council was happy to accept the reintroduction of a freedom of practice clause, but the standardising power of QA had become embedded in legislation.

To summarise, it can be suggested that developments in EBM and QA foster a tendency to the standardisation of practices. Although the focus has been within orthodox medicine, there has already been an impact on CAM practitioners within the established medical profession, and the impact will spread to CAM practitioners outside of medical practice.

Regulation and clinical freedom

Over the last 150 years there have been powerful forces unleashed that increasingly standardise medical practice and limit clinical freedom. The regulation of the medical profession through political processes culminated in the exclusion of many healing practices from state legitimacy. The imposition of higher educational standards gave doctors a greater status in relation to their rivals, eliminated certain classes of people from gaining a medical education, but also led to processes whereby those healing professions outside of established medicine set up similarly extensive periods of training in order to gain legitimacy. The modelling of these educational practices on mechanistic science cultivated conservative physicians. This process was further enhanced by the importation of statistical notions of normality into medicine, and the assumptions of standardised humans and standardised treatments excluded many therapeutic approaches from gaining the legitimacy of RCTs. Finally, science, regulation and education come together in the developing field of QA, which has the potential to ensure that qualified practitioners do not stray too far from the narrow paths of consensus medical practice. On the one hand, CAM can be seen as offering some resistance to the processes of standardisation. On the other hand, these medicines may be increasingly subject to the influences of standardisation.

The history of the medical profession shows how professional power was established but clinical freedom was assured. The state regulated the profession, but not the practice. Once granted such privileges, the medical profession could temper the practices of others. With the development of RCTs and their standardising assumptions, the medical profession had a new weapon to limit the claims of rivals. The CIC shows how outcomes were a mixture of traditional political lobbying and the imposition of medical views, leading to the limitation of chiropractic practice. However, the progressive use of QA means not only the regulation of the profession, but also increasingly the regulation of the practices. This use of QA is expanding to apply to all health professionals, not just the medical profession. Homogenised practitioners will increasingly use standardised procedures on a clientele conceptualised within a narrow set of norms.

The scenario depicted here is no doubt overstated. There was a proliferation of therapeutic practices offered to the public in the latter part of the twentieth century. The argument here is that there is a countervailing power to this proliferation, the power of regulation and standardisation of practices. This countervailing power is based around state concerns about variation in practice, the establishment of tighter norms of practice, and increasing the accountability of all practitioners to medical elites.

References

Allsop, J. and Mulcahy, L. (1996) *Regulating Medical Work: formal and informal Controls*, Buckingham: Open University Press.

Belgrave, M. (1985) *'Medical Men' and 'Lady Doctors': the making of a New Zealand profession, 1867–1941*, unpublished PhD thesis. Wellington: Victoria University of Wellington.

Berg, M. (1997) *Rationalizing Medical Work: decision-support techniques and medical practices*, Cambridge, MA: The Massachusetts Institute of Technology Press.

Berliner, H.S. (1984) 'Scientific medicine since Flexner', in Salmon, J. (ed.) *Alternative Medicines: popular and policy perspectives*, New York: Tavistock, pp. 30–56.

Boyd-Wilson, J. (1978) *To the Commission of Inquiry: paper to be presented by J.S. Boyd-Wilson in support of submissions by the New Zealand Medical Association and associated bodies*, Wellington: New Zealand Medical Association.

Clavarino, A. and Yates, P. (1995) 'Fear, faith or rational choice: understanding the users of alternative therapies', in Lupton, G. and Najman, J. (eds) *Sociology of Health and Illness: Australian Readings*, Melbourne: Macmillan, pp. 252–75.

Coburn, D. (1993a) 'Professional power in decline: medicine in a changing Canada', in Hafferty, F.W. and McKinlay, J.B. (eds) *The Changing Medical Profession: an international perspective*, New York: Oxford University Press pp. 92–103.

Coburn, D. (1993b) 'State authority, medical dominance, and trends in the regulation of the health professions: the Ontario case', *Social Science and Medicine* 37,2: 129–38.

Cole, D. (1985) 'Doctrinal deviance in New Zealand medical practice: some historical comments', *New Zealand Medical Journal* 98,782: 541–5.

Commission of Inquiry into Chiropractic (1979) *Chiropractic in New Zealand: Report of the Commission of Inquiry*, Wellington: Government Printer.

Coulter, H.L. (1973) *Divided Legacy: a history of the schism in medical thought. The patterns emerge: Hippocrates to Paracelsus*, Washington: Wehawken.

Curtis, S. and Taket, A. (1996) *Health and Societies: changing perspectives*, London: Arnold.

Daniels, S. (1992) 'The pragmatic management of error and the antecedents of disputes over the quality of medical care', in Dingwall, R. and Fenn, P. (eds) *Quality and Regulation in Health Care: international experiences*, London: Routledge pp. 112–40.

Dew, K. (1998) *Borderland Practices: validating and regulating alternative therapies in New Zealand*, unpublished PhD thesis, Wellington: Victoria University of Wellington.

Dew, K. (2000) 'Apostasy to orthodoxy: debates before a Commission of Inquiry into chiropractic', *Sociology of Health and Illness* 22,3: 1310–30.

Dew, K. (2001) 'Modes of practice and models of science in medicine', *Health: An Interdisciplinary Journal for the Study of Health, Illness and Medicine* 5,1: 93–111.

Duffy, J. (1979) *The Healers: a history of American medicine*, Chicago: University of Illinois Press.

Ellis, R. and Whittington, D. (1993) *Quality Assurance in Health Care: a handbook*, London: Edward Arnold.

Fisher, P. and Ward, A. (1994) 'Complementary medicine in Europe', *British Medical Journal* 309: 107–11.

Gow, P.J. (1981) 'Back pain management: groping for guidelines', *New Zealand Medical Journal* 93,686: 425–6.

Hacking, I. (1990) *The Taming of Chance*, Cambridge: Cambridge University Press.

Jost, T.S. (1992) 'Recent developments in medical quality assurance and audit', in Dingwall, R. and Fenn, P. (eds) *Quality and Regulation in Health Care: international experiences*, London: Routledge pp. 69–88.

Kaufman, M. (1971) *Homeopathy in America: the rise and fall of a medical heresy*, Baltimore: Johns Hopkins University Press.

Larkin, G. (1983) *Occupational Monopoly and Modern Medicine*. London: Tavistock.

Medical Practitioners Act (1995) Wellington: New Zealand Government.

New Zealand Medical Journal (1980a) 'NZMA proceedings of Council meeting, 12 December 1979, Wellington', 91,651: 114–116.

New Zealand Medical Journal (1980b) 'Back to it', 91,659: 345.

Osheron, S. and Amarasingham, L. (1981) 'The machine metaphor in medicine', in Mishler, E.G. (ed.) *Social Context of Health, Illness, and Patient Care*, Cambridge: Cambridge University Press.

Porter, T. (1995) *Trust in Numbers: the pursuit of objectivity in science and public life*, Princeton: Princeton University Press.

Rosenberg, C.E. (1992) *Explaining Epidemics and Other Studies in the History of Medicine*, Cambridge: Cambridge University Press.

Saks, M. (1994) 'The alternatives to medicine', in Gabe, J. and Kelleher, D. (eds) *Challenging Medicine*. London: Routledge, pp. 84–103.

Salmon, J. (1984) 'Introduction', in Salmon, J. (ed.) *Alternative Medicines: popular and policy perspectives*, New York: Tavistock, pp. 1–29.

Seale, C. (1993) 'The consumer voice', in Davey, B. and Popay, J. (eds) *Dilemmas in Health Care*. Buckingham: Open University Press, pp. 64–80.

Sigsworth, E.M. (1972) 'Gateways to death? Medicine, hospitals and mortality, 1700–1850', in Mathias, P. (ed.) *Science and Society 1600–1900*, London: Cambridge University Press, pp. 97–110.

Ward Report (1975) *Victorian Legislative Joint Select Committee on Osteopathy, Chiropractic and Naturopathy Report*.

Webb, Edwin (1977) *Chiropractic, Osteopathy, Homeopathy and Naturopathy*. Report of a Committee of Inquiry. Canberra: Acting Commonwealth Government Printer.

Waddington, I. (1977) 'General practitioners and consultants in early nineteenth-century England: the sociology of an intra-professional conflict', in Woodward, J. and Richards, D. (eds) *Health Care in Popular Medicine in Nineteenth Century England*, London: Croom Helm, pp. 164–88.

Willis, E. (1983) *Medical Dominance: the division of labour in Australian health-care*, Sydney: George Allen & Unwin.

Wilson, M. (1992) 'Towards a feminist jurisprudence in Aotearoa', in Du Plessis, Rosemary (ed.) *Feminist Voices: women's studies texts for Aotearoa/New Zealand*. Auckland: Oxford University Press.

Chapter 5

The corporatisation and commercialisation of CAM

Fran Collyer

Introduction

This chapter describes the market for Complementary and Alternative Medicine (CAM) and demonstrates its progression from a cottage industry to a mature market sector. A comparison is made between the historical reshaping of the CAM market and that of the orthodox healthcare sector, both of which have undergone significant marketisation. The chapter proposes that this marketisation process has been central to the integration of CAM within the mainstream healthcare sector, not just in Australia but internationally, and that the emerging integration between two formerly distinct markets has numerous implications, particularly for health policy and health system financing.

Among most Westernised, industrial societies, the majority of CAM practitioners have historically been small business operators, selling health services and healing aids in a competitive marketplace. In this, the history of CAM has not been dissimilar to that of the early orthodox practitioners. In contrast to orthodox medicine however, the state has not intervened in this market. CAM has generally been excluded from state support and financial subsidy, and it has not been granted a presence within public institutions. Also, CAM has survived within private clinics and centres that have often followed philanthropic, religious or spiritual objectives, though many have operated on a fee-for-service basis. These early CAM practitioners offered services in their own homes or from rented consulting rooms, some as family concerns and many as small, practitioner-owned businesses or partnerships. While the production of profit was essential for most if not all practitioners, entrepreneurial interests were often curtailed by alternative or competing objectives such as business autonomy, religion or philanthropy.

Increasingly however, as the end of the twentieth century drew near, CAM practitioners became employees of large companies, or employees or operators of nationwide franchises. And these businesses no longer offer purely CAM services: it is becoming decidedly more common to find an 'integrated' clinic bridging both allopathy and CAM, with practitioners trained in both paradigms. Paralleling this trend, and perhaps driving it, we also find that the many therapeutic products, equipment and devices used by these practitioners are increasingly manufactured and distributed by large national and multinational companies. Although vitamins and mineral supplements were the first CAM products to become 'mainstream' production items, and the vitamin market to be one of the first sectors of the CAM industry to become fully developed in countries such as Australia, other sectors have rapidly followed. It is now almost commonplace to find large national and multinational companies with business interests ranging fully across the health product spectrum: from the manufacture, distribution or sale of herbal remedies and Chinese medicine to high-tech, synthetic, designer drugs; from acupuncture needles and massage tables to high-technology diagnostic equipment; from the sale of health insurance to the provision of health services or practitioner training; and the ownership or management of retail outlets, hospitals, clinics and pathology laboratories. At the opening of the twenty-first century, CAM has finally become 'big business'.

A transformation in the orthodox healthcare system

The road CAM has followed from a 'cottage industry' to full global commercialisation and corporatisation has its similarities with the one taken by orthodox medicine. In Australia we have witnessed a remarkable transformation of the orthodox healthcare sector over the past two decades. This sector has altered from being a 'cottage industry' (composed of numerous small, owner-operated, independent private hospitals and medical practices, and dominated by many larger, public and not-for-profit hospitals), to a mature market sector. This dramatic shift began with the purchasing of 'chains' of private hospitals by large and diverse companies in the late 1970s, and it picked up pace in the early 1990s with the sale or contracting out of public hospitals to the private sector (Collyer 1997; White and Collyer 1998). These developments continued throughout the 1990s, with the increasing popularity for contracts with the private sector to build and/or run public (i.e. Medicare) hospitals, and the co-location of private hospitals adjacent to public hospitals (Collyer 1998). By the turn of the century this *marketisation* of the healthcare sector had shifted up a full gear. Moving beyond the provision of hospital services, these same companies have found new business opportunities by acquiring medical centres (White 2001); entering into contracts with government to deliver community health services such as drug and alcohol rehabilitation and veterans' services (Kelly 1995; Lyons 1997); and by acquiring allied health businesses (such as radiology, pathology and pharmacy) (Collyer and White 2001; Price 2001). These processes have been variously described elsewhere as vertical integration, corporatisation, privatisation and marketisation (see for example Collyer and White 2001).

CAM becomes part of the orthodox healthcare industry

While debates have raged in countries such as Australia, Britain and the USA over the impact of this restructuring for health policy and the financing of Medicare, the NHS and Medicaid, CAM has quietly yet steadily become part of mainstream corporate activity. Most patients leaving an orthodox pharmacy after having their prescription filled will be at least partially aware of the fact that a pharmaceutical company, probably a large and international one, produced the pills or lotion they now hold in their hands. And most would be able to recall at least a few of the names of these companies – perhaps Sigma, Glaxo-Welcome or Pfizer. But how many could bring to mind the names of the companies behind the alternative or complementary medicines they might also use? Among consumers, very little is known about these companies, despite the fact that most will admit to purchasing CAM therapies and consumers have increasingly returned to CAM products and practitioners over the past couple of decades. This shift represents a remarkable development, given the hegemony of orthodox medicine during the past century and a half, and it is a trend now evident in Australia, the USA, the UK and Europe (Eisenberg *et al.* 1998; Vincent and Furnham 1998). In Australia, the renewal of CAM has been particularly rapid. In 1993, 20 per cent of Australians visited a CAM practitioner and 49 per cent used CAM products (MacLennan *et al.* 1996). By the turn of the century, between 57 and 70 per cent of the population were using CAM (Gripper 1999; Russell 1999; Madden 2002).

Yet despite (or perhaps because of) the popularity of CAM, there is a prevailing view that CAM is somehow divorced from the world of commerce: that CAM services are not commercial transactions but altruistic exchanges associated with holistic notions of health whereby practitioners offer a more ethical and caring approach to individuals and their health needs; and that CAM products are more 'natural' and therefore safer than synthetic, high-technology products. These views are extremely common (see for example Coward 1989; Siahpush 1998; Singh and Franson 2001). They may be understood best as ideologies which obscure some of the 'less palatable' facts about CAM: the most unpalatable of which may be that this too is a highly profit-directed industry, with its fortunes rising and falling – not according to the integrity of the practitioner or their competency in keeping the consumer well – but on the price of shares, on clever takeovers and mergers, strategic joint ventures, on the timing and cost of new discoveries, on cost-cutting and downsizing, and on the effectiveness of corporate marketing campaigns.

The size of the CAM industry

The literature is replete with statements about the size of the CAM industry in Australia and elsewhere. For instance, it is stated that over-the-counter health products are currently worth $AU135bn worldwide, within which vitamin supplements alone are worth $AU49bn (Eakin 2000). In Australia in 1993, CAM services generated a turnover of about $AU480m, and $AU621m for medicines (MacLennan *et al.* 1996). Nearly one decade later, consumers were spending over $AU1.2bn per year on Chinese medicines alone (Owens 2001) and $AU800m per year on natural supplement products (ASX 2001). In fact, Australians are spending approximately twice as much on CAM as they are on orthodox pharmaceuticals (Gripper 1999; Macken 1999; Russell 1999), which is a little different from the USA, where consumers are spending similar amounts on alternative and mainstream products (Eisenberg *et al.* 1998).[1]

Definitional issues

But in making such statements about the size of the CAM industry, we meet an immediate definitional problem. How is the CAM industry constituted? Where are its borders? What distinguishes a CAM product or service from orthodox medicine? When estimates are made of the size of the CAM industry, what is included and excluded? Such questions are extraordinarily difficult to answer, primarily because this is a 'moving field': therapies and products are increasingly redefined as part of mainstream medical practice, and are quickly being assimilated into the mainstream healthcare industry. Moreover, definitions of CAM vary cross-culturally and across national boundaries (see Easthope *et al.* 2000). It is thus difficult to reach consensus over what might constitute a list of CAM services or products. Disagreements may occur over the inclusion of chiropractic or acupuncture as CAM, though perhaps there may be greater consensus over aromatherapy, naturopathy or iridology. When we look to the market and its diverse array of services and products, we may agree that mineral or herbal products are CAM, but should we also include 'functional confectionary' that might soothe a sore throat with lemon and honey? And should we also include the market for diet and nutritional foods? This market includes 'energy bars', soy-based meat alternatives for vegetarians, organic foods and products for individuals with allergies and food intolerances (for example, gluten-free flour or lactose-free milk). Currently the size of this market (globally) is $US31.7bn and growing at 11.3 per cent annually (see Harrison 2000). And should we not also consider as CAM the production of raw materials for making these products? For example, the gelatin capsules which are later filled with an active, therapeutic product; the growing of sage or tea tree; or the production of milk for the extraction of active compounds from which therapies can be made. This too is a rapidly growing area: the herbal medicine market for crude extracts alone is worth $US24bn per year worldwide (source: Pharmaction website). And consider also the possibility of including within our CAM market the manufacture of equipment and devices essential for the delivery of therapies. For example, there is a company in Victoria, Acuneeds Australia, that provides acupuncture needles, electrical stimulators, models, charts and books. Is this not also part of the CAM market? The definition can be complicated further. If devices and equipment are essential elements of the CAM industry, are not the systems of research and training, service delivery, health insurance, information technology, and financial management also fundamental components of the CAM industry?

CAM is often distinguished from scientific medicine by its unique epistemological and philosophical approach to health (see Coulter, Chapter 6). CAM is thought to be based upon 'the notion of the fundamental and integral unity of the body, the mind, and the spirit' (Salmon 1984: 8). The CAM approach to health emphasises self-responsibility, the building of a social identity and the accumulation of cultural assets. Orthodox or scientific medicine in contrast, is characterised as crudely materialist: disease is reducible to a disorder in an individual's biology that can be treated independently of social behaviour, social context and psychological state. However, these contrasting orientations toward the understanding of health and the nature of reality offer insufficient explanation for the historical marginalisation of CAM products, services and practitioners. After all, the distinction between CAM and orthodox medicine is a fairly recent one in historical terms. It arose only with the twin developments of scientific medicine and the professionalisation of orthodox practitioners, a process most significant during the nineteenth century when there was a plethora of competing theories of health and illness. While different philosophical orientations were present, and continue to be so, the importance of these ideas rests largely on how they have been taken up in practice and institutionalised. In particular, how they have been used ideologically to secure the interests of one group over those of another. After all, ideas alone, no matter how interesting or compelling, are rarely sufficient to bring about social change (Cohen 1968: 179). In other words, ideas have *causal* significance in the process of social change only when they are realised in social practice. Thus it is most important to understand how these alternative conceptions of health have come to shape the way healthcare is practised, and how they might have shaped the healthcare market, bringing about a division between CAM and orthodox medical products and services.

One explanation for the division in the marketplace is that CAM's epistemological framework led to a form of practice in the nineteenth century which was less amenable than other forms of healing to market commodification. The form of knowledge that became dominant was the 'medical model': a form of knowledge most compatible with dominant class interests, and so fostered by this class (Willis 1983: 24). This compatibility between the medical model used by orthodox practitioners and the class system can be explained by the fact that the medical model is built upon a fundamental Cartesian dualism between mind and body, subject and object. Only from within this epistemological stance can a medical knowledge emerge in which illness is defined as a dysfunction of particular body parts that require repair or replacement: as if the body were a machine. And only this epistemology can give rise to a form of medical practice in which there is a hierarchy between healer and patient, requiring and, indeed, necessitating objective intervention and a passive submission, rather than a mutual interaction between equals during the healing process (for further discussion see Inglis 1981: 266).

In contrast, alternative epistemologies produce very different models of illness and forms of healthcare organisation. For example, if one assumes a Kantian, dialectical response to nature and culture, both participants (doctor and patient) are active, interpreting actors, not an observer and a passive agent; and health is a balance or harmony between nature and culture, not a battle between the two in which nature must be 'conquered'. Yet history shows us that only highly interventionist and hierarchical forms of medicine became commercially lucrative and amenable to the expansion of capital during the nineteenth century. This idea is encapsulated in Willis's explanation for the compatibility between capitalism and allopathic medicine. He suggests that forms of medicine that did not become dominant conformed to an 'Individualist' mode of practice, while the allopathic group conformed to a 'Corporatist' mode, and it was the latter group that became dominant. While both groups originally had a similar mode of practice (a form of small, petit bourgeois production where the therapies and instruments can be located within a bag or basket), only the dominant group was incorporated within the intensive production model of capitalism in which there is a development and exchange of expensive technologies and the support of large, central institutions (Willis 1983: 22).

Thus, we can see that a fracturing of the healthcare system was created, where the form of prominent healing was that which primarily took only the organic nature of illness into account and offered therapies which were readily commodified as pharmaceutical preparations or other technological forms of intervention. It is not difficult to understand that the much higher potential for profit of scientific medicine ensured that it was supported by class interests and was also provided with the support of the state, the scientific institutions, philanthropic foundations (such as Rockefeller) and importantly, the medical schools themselves (see Berliner 1984: 33–5; Eisenberg *et al.* 1993).

The 150-year marginalisation of alternative health knowledges, CAM practitioners, and their products reached its zenith when world production systems were in high gear and when public confidence in science and orthodox medicine were greatest: during the 1950s to 1970s. During this period, the healthcare industry was cleaved into two distinct markets. On the one hand were large national and international companies producing ethical, 'high-tech' pharmaceuticals, medical devices and equipment, large publicly funded institutions for research and the training of practitioners, and practitioners with high salaries and well-defined career progression. On the other hand was a small cottage industry turning out aromatic oils, herbal mixtures and iridology charts, much smaller and private institutions for education and training, little formalised research, and often unpaid or underpaid practitioners with no state or professional recognition of their skill or expertise. By the beginning of the twenty-first century, this industry has changed dramatically.

A snapshot of the CAM industry in Australia

It is possible to draw a rough picture of the CAM industry in Australia if fine distinctions and definitions are put to one side. Rather, relying strongly on the terminology of market analysts and journalists, we find that while the healthcare market as a whole is worth about $AU50bn (including forty-four health funds, 1,500 hospital and day surgeries, 36,000 clinicians, plus manufacturers and suppliers of drugs, equipment and services: see ASX 2002), the CAM market is apparently much smaller at between $AU1–2bn (Macken 1999; *Courier Mail* 2000; Moynihan 2000). However, it is important to note that such estimates generally focus on the production, manufacture and sale of products, excluding the markets for research, training, services and insurance.

In the manufacturing sector, there are nine sizeable companies that produce CAM products and are listed on the Australian Stock Exchange (ASX). Of these, six have listed only fairly recently, several are in the top 100 performing companies, and one was placed in administration in December 2001 (Cottee Health). Many of these manufacturing companies produce vitamins, mineral and nutritional supplements (a large and well-established component of the CAM market) but others manufacture products that are less orthodox, such as homoeopathic remedies, Chinese medicines (for example, Analytica), and medicines based on the derivatives of plants or animals (such as the oestrogen replacement therapies manufactured by Novogen). However, this list of CAM companies could easily be expanded to include similar manufacturers not listed on the ASX, such as Cardia (and its subsidiaries Natural Pharmacy, Herbworx and Transherbal) or ASX listed companies that mainly produce orthodox products but have some association with CAM, such as AMRAD with its extensive

Table 5.1 CAM manufacturing companies listed on the ASX

Listing	Company
1	Pan Pharmaceuticals
2	Faulding, Cenovis, Bullivant (Mayne Group)
3	Clover
4	Blackmores
5	Herbs of Gold, Vita Health (Vita Life Sciences)
6	Novogen
7	Modern Chinese Medicine (Analytica)
8	Pharmaction, Biologic, BETA (Cottee Health)
9	Anadis

library of natural substances, each potentially a pharmaceutical drug. More-over, if over-the-counter products such as plant-based hand lotions are also taken into consideration, then the net can be thrown wider to include companies such as Amcal and Guardian (controlled by Sigma), and Soul Pattison (controlled by Australian Pharmaceutical Industries). And if the production of natural, raw materials is included in the definition of CAM, then it will also encompass companies such as Australian Plantations (which produces and exports tea tree oil), Aroma Australis, Sunspirit Aromatherapy and Essential Health (producing natural plant oils, herbs and herbal extracts).

The mainstreaming of the CAM industry

The evidence for the mainstreaming of CAM can be found in various locations such as the training and research sectors, where large public insti-tutions have begun to conduct research and offer courses in CAM. This is the case in many countries, including the USA (see Meadows 2001) and Australia (see Leys 2000; Pachacz 2001). It can also be found in the inclusion of CAM within mainstream health insurance packages. Insurers are more likely to do this in the USA than in Australia, as at least eleven US states mandate the inclusion of chiropractic (see Rauber 1998). How-ever, even in Australia, where funds are not allowed to accredit practi-tioners and where there are no Health Maintenance Organisations (HMOs) as such, many insurance companies are using CAM as a marketing device to attract healthy (and therefore higher profit) customers (see Bye 1997; Macken 1999; Benko 2000).

Perhaps one of the most interesting areas of mainstreaming has occurred in CAM services, which has been the slowest sector to leave its cottage industry status behind. Many CAM practitioners, such as naturopaths, work in private clinics but, increasingly, they are being employed by corporations such as vitamin or pharmaceutical companies (Leys 2000), in corporately owned 'integrated' or 'holistic' clinics, and in the growing numbers of CAM research and training centres attached to universities and colleges (see Phelan 1997). Mainstreaming can also be seen in the way increasing numbers of GPs are now referring patients to CAM practitioners (Moynihan 2000) and are themselves becoming multi-skilled, using chiropractic and acupuncture therapies as part of their repertoire. This kind of mainstreaming is a form of co-option, where the practitioners use the techniques and equipment without adopting the alternative knowledge base of CAM. A similar process is occurring among a range of other health workers (including nurses and the allied professions) and in many conventional Australian hospitals, both private and public.

In some cases this co-option of CAM is formalised into the organisational structure, and the hospital or clinic is marketed as an 'integrated' institution, offering a wide range of CAM and non-CAM services. The sixty-bed private Swinburne University Hospital in Victoria is of this type. A variation on this is found among institutions which offer co-located CAM services marketed as holistic or integrated health centres. An example can be found at the Shellharbour Private Hospital, south of Sydney, which has set up a one-stop medical complex offering both CAM and non-CAM services and products next door to the hospital (*Illawarra Mercury* 2000). To date however, integrated clinics have not attracted major corporate interest in Australia, and there has not been a large-scale 'chaining' of CAM or integrated clinics under one corporate umbrella – as has occurred with hospitals, pathology laboratories, radiology and GP medical centres. This situation contrasts with the USA, where over 10 per cent of hospitals and up to 65 per cent of HMOs are now providing alternative medicine, where there are many hospital-sponsored integrated clinics offering all forms of CAM from hypnosis to relaxation (Bellandi 1999; Meadows 2001), and where chains of branded, integrated clinics have emerged (Thompson 2000).

Within the manufacturing sector, mainstreaming is also in evidence. Here it can be found in the changing production practices of manufacturers. The Australian case can be used as an example, as it is far from unique. Where once manufacturers produced either CAM or orthodox products, today only three of the nine listed manufacturing companies exclusively produce CAM products (Blackmores, Clover and Anadis), and one of these (Anadis) is on the verge of extending into pharmaceutical production. This general mixing of CAM and non-CAM manufacturing, together with the very size of these companies (for they are now comparable to firms that produce orthodox products) indicates clearly that in regard to manufacturing, CAM no longer forms a distinct market sector.

A similar level of mainstreaming has occurred in the distribution and retailing of CAM products. In Australia, the wholesale distribution market

Table 5.2 The drug wholesale and retail sectors

	Wholesale (%)	Retail (%)	Chemist chains
Sigma	30	20	Amcal, Russells and Guardian
API	27	24	Soul Pattison, Chemworld, Pharmacist Advice and API Healthcare
Mayne (Faulding)	38	11	Terry White, The Medicine Shoppe, Life, Healthsense and ChemMart

Source: from figures supplied by Field (1998)

for pharmaceuticals is shared largely between three companies: Sigma, API and Mayne (see Table 5.2). These companies are now also involved in the distribution of CAM-related products. Mainstreaming has also occurred in the retailing sector. Two to three decades ago CAM products were largely sold in specialised alternative health shops. Today most chemists stock CAM products, and supermarkets are increasingly an outlet (Weisner 1998; ASX 2000; for the UK figures, see *Mintel Report* 2001). In Australia this shift has occurred in parallel with a significant corporatisation of the pharmaceutical retail sector. Although drug distributors cannot purchase retail pharmacies, they can form buying groups, controlling the supply of products to individual pharmacies and pharmacy chains. The three main drug distributors, Sigma, API and Mayne, together control over 95 per cent of the wholesale drug market, and 55 per cent of the retail sector. Many of the pharmacies controlled by these companies sell both CAM and non-CAM products, with Amcal (Sigma) and Soul Pattison (API) stocking Blackmore's products and the Mayne group stocking the Mayne products Cenovis and Bullivants. In fact, the latest trend has been the setting up of a branded natural medicine counter within the pharmacies themselves, in direct competition with the healthfood stores (see Cosslett 1999).

The formation of a CAM industry through merger and acquisition

In Australia, much of the mainstreaming of the CAM industry has been accomplished by mergers and acquisitions rather than by companies altering their manufacturing processes or internally expanding their product range through R&D. For example, Cottee Health International (formerly Biologic International) was a suspended waste processor company. It acquired Cottee International in March 2001 and, in doing so, became a manufacturer and supplier of CAM products, including dietary supplements and natural personal care products. In October 2001, Cottee International acquired Pharmaction Manufacturing, which manufactures OTC, prescription products and natural therapeutics. In acquiring Pharmaction, Cottee also gained a 75 per cent ownership of BETA, which produces soy-based natural pharmaceuticals and purifies bio-actives from herbal components.

A second example is the Mayne Group, which started out as a transport and logistics company (Mayne Nickless), but in 1986 it bought into the hospital sector with the purchase of a 20 per cent stake in a Newcastle-based chain of five hospitals. In 1988 it gained a 51 per cent holding in the Hospitals of Australia Trust, and in 1991 with the purchase of the US company, Hospital Corporation of Australia, Mayne became the largest operator of private hospital beds in Australia. It has maintained this position, but has expanded (through acquisition) into pathology, radiology and medical practices. In 2001 it acquired FH Faulding, a drug manufacturer that had itself acquired the CAM businesses of Bullivants and Cenovis. With these acquisitions, Mayne has secured its place alongside Blackmores as one of the two biggest manufacturers and distributors of CAM products in Australia.

A third example is Vita Life Sciences, a Melbourne-based company which listed on the ASX in 2000. Vita Life has several divisions, including Vita Medical (formerly Tetley Medical) which has 78 per cent of the nuclear imaging market in Australia; Vita Pharma which, through joint ventures with German and Chinese companies, manufactures prescription pharmaceuticals; and Vita Health. This latter division was formed through the acquisition of the company Herbs of Gold in April 2001 (ASX 2001). Herbs of Gold had a well-established brand of 142 herbal and health supplement products on the Australian market. As a result of this acquisition, Vita Health now produces both CAM and OTC products for the Australian and Asian markets.

Many other companies have entered the CAM market through acquisitions and mergers, and few CAM companies have not engaged in this activity. One that stands apart is Blackmores, a company still guided by a Blackmores family member and selling its products under its own label in natural health food stores, pharmacies and supermarket chains. It is one of the few which manufactures its own products (rather than using contract manufacturing), conducts research and product development (often in conjunction with universities), and has its own established brand name.

The fact that the Australian CAM manufacturing industry has been formed through acquisition and merger is significant. It is important for a small economy to have large companies with the economies of scale to enter the global marketplace, and it would be difficult to prevent acquisitive behaviour given that it is, after all, a fundamental and often forgotten feature of competition: companies will act to eliminate competition wherever possible, often by swallowing competitors. Nevertheless, acquisitive behaviour and the elimination of smaller companies can be quite harmful to an economy, as they reduce the diversity of the marketplace, increase the likelihood of monopoly and reduce innovation (because it is the smaller firms which are significant innovators while larger companies tend to use acquisition rather than in-house R&D as a means of technology transfer). In addition, mergers and acquisitions are costly activities which do not of themselves give rise to innovation or new product development: in other words, they add little to the production of goods and services. In countries where the state subsidises or pays for healthcare services, mergers and acquisitions raise the cost of healthcare to governments. In private health-care markets they raise the costs to other third-party providers, consumers and patients. The Institute for Health and Socio-Economic Policy in Canada (IHSP 2001) recently reported on the impact of the modification of the Anti-Trust legislation in 1995 to allow mergers and acquisitions in the healthcare industry. This legislative change was initiated on the pre-sumption that total healthcare spending would be reduced by assisting the healthcare industry to grow and achieve economies of scale. The Institute found that, contrary to expectations, the impact of mergers and acquisitions was to increase total health spending. Mergers and acquisitions, particularly in the pharmaceutical sector, have enabled the industry to increase prices, put pressure on hospitals to reduce staffing, and reduce patient access to healthcare services (IHSP 2001: 16, 18).

Vertical integration and CAM

The incorporation of CAM into orthodox medical practice through the multi-skilling of doctors and other health workers, the development of inte-grated clinics and hospitals, the introduction of CAM into the mainstream training and research institutions, and the addition of CAM products into orthodox manufacturing and distribution systems, have all become features of the healthcare sector during the last decade. Vertical integration too has become commonplace. In this process, companies build or purchase several related businesses (such as pathology laboratories or hospitals) and capitalise on their investment in one product or service area by 'capturing' the referrals to other parts of the system (see Collyer and White 2001). The ownership of several related businesses ensures that companies can channel customers toward their other businesses,[2] drive up demand for services, and form strategic alliances to increase market share and minimise costs and tax. This activity is easily demonstrated with an example from the orthodox health sector where a group of twenty GPs, placed under one corporate umbrella, generate about $AU50m in flow-on health expenditure to other business areas such as drugs, pathology, diagnostics, surgery and hospital care (Price 2001). Empirical studies show practitioners are still a very important means of product distribution (especially for homoeopathic products, see ASX 1998), and that the sale of CAM products increases by

25 per cent amongst individuals who visit practitioners (MacLennan *et al.* 1996). Thus, it makes sense for companies that are producing products to have a means to encourage consumers to visit practitioners so that they can increase sales. This integration process is not unique to Australia. The 'chaining' of hospitals in America was described over two decades ago by Relman as the formation of a new medical-industrial complex (1980: 996–7), and there are clear signs of similar corporate strategies being implemented in the UK (Pollock *et al.* 2001).

What is new in the healthcare systems of these countries is the addition of CAM services and products, allowing the development of a network of referrals between CAM and non-CAM health services. In the Australian market, the vertical integration strategies of the corporate sector have only just begun to include CAM. Many of the major biotech (pharmaceutical) companies (such as CSL) do not manufacture CAM products, and many of the hospital or nursing home companies (such as Ramsay, Healthscope and Moran) focus on management and service delivery and either do not engage in the manufacturing or distribution of healthcare products or only manufacture orthodox pharmaceuticals (for example, Sonic Healthcare and its subsidiary SciGen). Nevertheless, there is an increasing level of vertical integration which incorporates both CAM and non-CAM products and services. One example of this is Vita Life Sciences. This company manufactures CAM products such as vitamins, supplements, healthfoods and functional confectionary, as well as nutraceuticals, and registered and OTC pharmaceuticals. It also produces diagnostic medical equipment and is a large player in the radiology and nuclear imaging market. A second example is Australian Pharmaceutical Industries, which operates a large hospital supply business (via its acquisition of Hospital Supplies of Australia in October 2000), is a major player in the wholesale pharmaceutical and retail distribution business, offers financial and marketing services to pharmacy retailers through its subsidiary API Finance Ltd., has a developing interest in building information technology systems for pharmacies, and has a small manufacturing business through its acquisition of Soul Pattison. A third example is Mayne Health. This company is the largest player in the hospitals and pathology markets, has a significant interest in the general practice market and in radiology, is a major wholesaler for drugs, has a significant retail interest in pharmacies (selling both CAM and orthodox products), and is a major distributor of hospital supplies. In addition, it has a manufacturing interest in both CAM and orthodox products through its acquisition of Bullivant's Natural Health Products and Cenovis. These few examples indicate that, although Australian companies have increasingly engaged in vertical integration in the healthcare industry since the 1990s, it is only very recently that CAM services and products have begun to be included.

The impact of the mainstreaming of CAM

CAM and orthodox medicine have travelled similar routes from *cottage industry* to *corporatisation*, but the time it has taken for their respective journeys has varied remarkably. The mainstreaming of CAM has finally ended a 150-year fracturing of the marketplace, in which past restrictions to either CAM or orthodox medicine have dissolved for both practitioners and corporations. The mainstreaming of CAM at the turning of the century is a healing of this fracture, a reintegration of the healthcare market into one, new, strategically powerful industry.

Yet it needs to be said that this reintegration of CAM has occurred only at the level of products, services and techniques. It is very clearly a co-option of CAM, not an amalgamation of philosophies or knowledges. There is little evidence that the mainstreaming of CAM represents an under-mining of the hegemonic medical model of illness, nor is it a challenge to scientific practice and the major institutions. This mainstreaming process is neither an equal partnership between the two systems nor a reformulation of the health system. It is instead a revitalisation of the orthodox market system, in which clever marketing and acquisition strategies have been used to ensure that CAM is made amenable to a high production, high profit system, enabling companies to expand into new product and service areas and extending their reach beyond the established boundaries of the healthcare system.

There are at least two important consequences of the mainstreaming of CAM. The first of these is the inevitable loss of autonomy for CAM practitioners within the healthcare system. Prior to reintegration, CAM practitioners were primarily small-business owners, a status they shared with early orthodox practitioners. When orthodox practitioners began to take up salaried positions within private and public enterprises, there was a decline in the autonomy of the medical profession as a whole (Haug 1975; McKinlay 1982; White and Collyer 1997; Collyer and White 2001; White 2001). Despite the fact that CAM has finally been remodelled into the 'corporatist' mode of practice, with its products and services mainstreamed into the healthcare market, and its research and training activities taken up by the major public institutions, the mainstreaming of CAM has occurred at the wrong historical moment for a strengthening of practitioner autonomy. At this point in history, there is a decline in the power of the state over the healthcare system. Unlike orthodox medicine, which professionalised during the nineteenth century with the support of the state (and at a time when the state itself was increasing in strength), CAM practitioners are regaining public credibility and expanding their services at a time of declining healthcare budgets and state withdrawal from the policy arena.

This withdrawal of the state is most evident in the USA and Australia, though Britain has not been free of pro-marketisation policies. In the USA, it is evident in the introduction of a corporately controlled, managed care system which has driven down quality and reduced clinical autonomy (Light 1993; Ginzberg 1999). In Australia, the national health insurance system (introduced in 1972) ensured some state control over health policy, planning and financing, even though it is an essentially fee-for-service system designed to accommodate practitioners as independent small-business operators.[3] However, the introduction of an American styled, corporately controlled, managed care system became possible after 1995 with the introduction of legislation to allow third-party contracting. Various companies have taken up this opportunity. For example, the insurance company AXA now has more than half the 8,000 specialists in Victoria and South Australia under contract and is selectively tendering with hospitals that meet its cost and service guidelines (Uren 2001). This legislation, and policies which have encouraged marketisation, have significantly increased the role of corporations in the healthcare sector, and reduced the long-standing role of public institutions to set and maintain standards. One of its many casualties is a reduction in the autonomy of doctors and other healthcare workers.

A second important outcome of mainstreaming is the escalation of health-care costs for both consumers and the state. There is already sufficient evidence that, at the national level, market-based healthcare systems have higher costs than those which are publicly delivered and financed, and that the intensification of private sector involvement in healthcare offers little longterm benefit to the nations themselves. This holds true in the American situation (Lewin *et al.* 1981; Pattison and Katz 1983; Himmelstein *et al.* 1999), the Australian situation (White and Collyer 1997; Duckett and Jackson 2000; SCARC 2000, submission 41; Collyer and White 2001), and in the British (Pollock *et al.* 2000). Any international comparison of health costs per capita will immediately reveal the disadvantages of a market system, with the USA being crippled with rising costs of 12.4 per cent of GDP, Australia with its mixed system holding fairly steady at 8.2 per cent, Norway at 7.4 per cent, and the UK with its publicly funded and largely publicly provided NHS the lowest at 6.2 per cent (Nathan 1997: 14).

With CAM added to the national healthcare system through the process of mainstreaming, the consequence will be a further escalation of costs because this is essentially a market strategy to expand market share and drive up demand. Although the integration of CAM into these healthcare systems may bring some benefits to consumers in the form of more inclusive services, increased knowledge about techniques and therapies, and perhaps more testing and regulation of CAM therapies and products, mainstreaming can only raise costs to consumers, third-party contributors and govern-ments. After all, mainstreaming is fundamentally a market strategy. It is an

aspect of vertical integration and it is created out of the process of commodification of healthcare products and services. Mainstreaming is clearly
about profit. It bears little relation to the enhancement of well-being, patient
safety, altruism or the curing of disease.

Notes

1 This difference can easily be explained by the fact that in Australia only orthodox pharmaceuticals are subsidised by the government through the Pharmaceutical Benefit Scheme, and this keeps the direct costs to the patient low by
   world standards.
2 In Australia this is particularly important because patients cannot seek out a
   specialist or ask a laboratory to perform a diagnostic test; they must have a
   referral from a general practitioner.
3 Medibank was introduced by the Whitlam government in 1972. It has undergone several revisions, including a change of name to Medicare. This National
   Insurance system provides all citizens and permanent residents with free or
   heavily subsidised healthcare services (at the point of service), irrespective of
   whether they attend a public or privately owned health hospital or clinic. Other
   aspects of the Medicare system provide funds for the construction and maintenance of hospitals, and subsidise the purchase of pharmaceuticals and other
   services such as radiology and pathology. Medicare is partially funded through
   a levy on taxpayers (the Medicare levy). The majority of the funding for healthcare services comes from general tax revenue. For the first couple of decades,
   this system ensured high-income earners paid a higher levy. This is no longer
   the case as high-income earners can now receive a reduction in their Medicare
   levy if they join a private health insurance fund.

References

ASX (1998) *Letter to Shareholders – Progress Report on Current Status of Company*.
   Statement from Medicine Quantale Ltd., Australian Stock Exchange announce-
   ment, 20 August 2:02:06 pm.
ASX (2000) *Results of AGM*. Statement from Blackmores Ltd., Australian Stock
   Exchange announcement, 29 March 12:57:01 pm.
ASX (2001) *Acquisition of Herbs of Gold*. Statement from Vita Life Sciences Ltd.,
   Australian Stock Exchange announcement, 19 March 9:28:52 am.
ASX (2002) *Healthscope Signing Gives THELMA a National Hospital Base*.
   Australian Stock Exchange announcement, 14 January 10:38:52 am.
Bellandi, D. (1999) 'AHA venture taps alternative medicine', *Modern Healthcare*
   27 September, 2.
Benko, L. (2000) 'Alternative medicine cuts costs as therapy', *Modern Healthcare*
   4 December, 30: 50.
Berliner, H.S. (1984) 'Scientific medicine since Flexner' in Salmon, W. (ed.) *Alterna-
   tive Medicines: popular and policy perspectives*, London: Tavistock, pp. 30–56.
Bye, C. (1997) 'Funds now willing to toss up a few more alternatives', *Sun Herald*
   12 July, 72.
Cohen, P. (1968) *Modern Social Theory*, London: Heinemann.

Collyer, F.M. (1997) 'The Port Macquarie Base Hospital: privatisation and the public purse', *Just Policy* 10, June: 27–39.

Collyer, F.M. (1998) 'Privatisation and Australian hospitals' *Health Issues* (Melbourne: Health Issues Centre), September: 56: 12–14.

Collyer, F.M. and White, K.N. (2001) *Corporate Control of Healthcare in Australia*, Discussion paper no. 42: Australia Institute, Australian National University.

Cosslett, G. (1999) 'Fighting for the future', *Sydney Morning Herald* 24 March, 23.

Courier Mail (2000) 'Life's ill effects fixed naturally', Brisbane: 29 July, C24.

Coward, R. (1989) *The Whole Truth: the myth of alternative health*, London: Faber & Faber.

Duckett, S. and Jackson, T. (2000) 'The new health insurance rebate: an inefficient way of assisting public hospitals', *Medical Journal of Australia* 172: 439–42.

Eakin, J. (2000) 'Pan to cash in on vitamin bug', *Sydney Morning Herald* 20 July.

Easthope, G., Tranter, B. and Gill, G. (2000) 'General Practitioner's attitudes toward complementary therapies', *Social Science and Medicine* 51,10: 1555–61.

Eisenberg, D.M., Kessler, R.C., Foster, C., Norloc, F.E., Calkins, D.R. and Delbanco, T.L. (1993) 'Unconventional medicine in the United States', *New England Journal of Medicine* 328: 246–52.

Eisenberg, D.M., Davis, R.B. , Ettner, S.L., Appel, S., Wilkey, S., Van Rompey, M. and Kessler, R.C. (1998) 'Trends in alternative medicine use in the United States, 1990–1997', *JAMA* 289, 18:1569–75.

Field, N. (1998) 'Chemistry of the drug business', *Australian Financial Review* 17 July, 54.

Ginzberg, E. (1999) 'The uncertain future of managed care', *The New England Journal of Medicine* 340(2), 14 January, 144–6.

Gripper, A. (1999) 'What's the alternative?', *Sydney Morning Herald* 22 November.

Harrison, J. (2000) 'UniLever joins other food giants scrambling to get healthy', *Mergers & Acquisitions* June, 35,6: 19.

Haug, M.R. (1975) 'The deprofessionalisation of everyone?', *Sociological Focus* 8: 197–213.

Himmelstein, D.U., Woolhandler, S., Hellander, I. and Wolfe, S. (1999) 'Quality of care in investor-owned vs not-for-profit HMOs', *The Journal of the American Medical Association* 282(2), 14 July, 159–63.

Illawarra Mercury (2000) 'One-stop medical shop on the way', 13 July, 41.

Inglis, B. (1981) *The Diseases of Civilisation*, London: Granada Publishing.

IHSP (2001) *'Big Pharma': mergers, drug costs and health caregiver staffing ratios*, Institute for Health and Socio-Economic Policy, Canada: Orinda.

Kelly, R. (1995) 'Privatising public health', *Just Policy* 3 June, 26–32.

Lewin, L., Derzon, R. and Margulies, R. (1981) 'Investor-owned and non-profits differ in economic performance', *Hospitals* 1 July, 52–8.

Leys, N. (2000) 'Paydirt', *Sydney Morning Herald* 12 February, 126.

Light, D. (1993) 'Escaping the traps of postwar Western medicine', *European Journal of Public Health* 3(4): 281–9.

Lyons, M. (1997) 'Contracting for care: how much is stere and is it the eay to go?', *Contracting For Care: Third Sector Review* 3, Special Issue: 205–25.

Macken, J. (1999) 'A healthy alternative', *Australian Financial Review* 2 March, 14.

McKinlay, J.B. (1982) 'Toward the proletarianisation of physicians' in Derber, C. and G.K. Hall (eds) *Professionals As Workers,* Boston.

MacLennan, A.H., Wilson, D.H. and Taylor, A.W. (1996) 'Prevalence and cost of alternative medicine in Australia', *Lancet* 347, 2: 569–73.

Madden, J. (2002) 'Natural becomes respectable', *The Australian*, health supplement, 13 March, 8.

Meadows, S. (2001) 'Kinder, gentler clinics', *Newsweek* 26 February, 52.

Mintel Report (2001) 'Complementary medicine', Online. Available HTTP: http://www.mintel.com

Moynihan, R. (2000) 'It's only natural', *Australian Financial Review* 8 April.

Nathan, S. (1997) 'Managed care or managed scare?', *Consuming Interest* Spring 73: 12–15.

Owens, S. (2001) 'Pointed message', *Australian Financial Review* 6 January.

Pachacz, M. (2001) 'New healthy alternative', *Shares* 1 April, 40.

Pattison, R. and Katz, H. (1983) 'Investor-owned and not-for-profit hospitals', *New England Journal of Medicine* 309: 347–53.

Pharmaction. Online. Available: http://www.biopharmalink.com/companies/1645htm

Phelan, A. (1997) 'Culture cure', *Sydney Morning Herald* Supplement 20 October, 1.

Pollock, A., Shaoul, J., Rowland, D. and Player, S. (2001) *Why It Matters Whether the Public Sector or the For-Profit Private Sector Delivers Key Public Services,* London: Health Policy and Health Services Research Unit, School of Public Policy, University College London.

Price, G. (2001) 'Firms fight for $2.7bn in doctor's fees', *The Australian* 16 July, 10.

Rauber, C. (1998) 'Open to alternatives', *Modern Healthcare* 7 September, 28(36): 50(1).

Relman, A. (1980) 'The new medical-industrial complex', *New England Journal of Medicine* 303: 963–70.

Russell, L. (1999) 'There's no alternative to good medicine', *Business Review Weekly* 5 November.

Salmon, W. (1984) 'Introduction' in Salmon, W. (ed), *Alternative Medicines: popular and policy perspectives,* London: Tavistock, pp. 1–29.

SCARC (Senate Community Affairs Reference Committee) (2000) *Healing Our Hospitals,* Australian Parliament. Online. Available HTTP: http://www.aph.gov.au/senate/committee/

Siahpush, M. (1998) 'Postmodern values, dissatisfaction with conventional medicine and popularity of alternative therapies', *Journal of Sociology* 34: 58–70.

Singh, S. and Franson, D. (2001) 'UK gets the urge to go herbal', *Marketing Week* 16 August, 34–5.

Thompson, E. (2000) 'The alternative model', *Modern Health Care* 15 May, 30: 26.

Uren, D. (2001) 'Health funds wield business end of the scalpel', *The Australian* 3 March, 48.

Vincent, C. and Furnham, A. (1998) *Complementary Medicine: a research perspective,* Chichester: Wiley.

Weisner, D. (1998) *Alternative Medicine: a guide for patients and health practitioners in Australia,* Melbourne: Kangaroo Press.

White, K.N. (2001) 'What's happening in general practice?', *Annual Review of Health Social Sciences* 10.

White, K.N. and Collyer, F.M. (1997) 'To market to market: corporatisation, privatisation and hospital costs', *Australian Health Review* July 20(2): 13–25.

White, K.N. and Collyer, F.M. (1998) 'Health care markets in Australia: ownership of the private hospital sector', *International Journal of Health Services* 28(3): 487–510.

Willis, E. (1983) *Medical Dominance,* Australia: George Allen & Unwin.

Part III

Boundary contestation in the workplace

Chapter 6

Integration and paradigm clash

The practical difficulties of integrative medicine

Ian Coulter

Introduction

Despite all the concerns in orthodox medicine about complementary and alternative medicine (CAM), it is clear that a major paradigm shift is also occurring within medicine itself. Within a very short period of time, medicine has moved from outright hostility to CAM to acknowledging its existence and finally co-operating with, and embracing, CAM. Increasingly, medicine is incorporating CAM into medical education and practice. Furthermore, this paradigm is increasingly being identified as 'integrative medicine'. This chapter will explore the challenge posed by trying to integrate two paradigms that hold fundamentally contradictory metaphysical beliefs, and differing philosophies, about health and healthcare. The chapter will draw on Thomas Kuhn's (1962) work on paradigms to explore this problem.

Metaphysics and science

Agassi (1964) has proposed that metaphysics play the dominant role in determining which scientific problems within any given period will be engaged with by the scientists, a role given to paradigms in Kuhn's (1962) theory. Metaphysics are broad generalisations about the nature of the world and are usually ontological (about the ultimate nature of reality). Unlike theories that try to make sense of observations, metaphysics are a priori in that they provide schemes in terms of which reality can be approached before we even begin to think about theory. Examples of metaphysics in science include mechanism, dualism, realism, idealism, materialism and reductionism. These are all fundamental presuppositions whose truth or falsehood cannot be established empirically through observation. They are also fundamental in the sense that the purpose of research done under their guidance is not to question or test these assumptions. To this extent, they are the taken-for-granted guidelines for investigation. If they are challenged, it will be through appeal to an alternative metaphysics.

So, for example, Descartes challenges the extreme notion of mechanism, and rescues mechanism by establishing a dualism to deal with the order of the mind. Current chaos theory challenges the metaphysic of determinacy.

Major metaphysical questions still haunt science (Watkins 1958). Wartofsky (1967) has suggested that the best way to think of metaphysics is to see them as a heuristic in science, as devices that are either useful or not useful rather than as true or not true. Metaphysics, therefore, is that branch of philosophy that makes explicit and critiques a priori assumptions (Kekes 1973).

The metaphysical systems underlying most of biomedicine, that is, mechanism and reductionism, may be criticised on numerous grounds and are now being challenged as the appropriate philosophical grounding for allopathic medicine, but they did give rise to a highly successful research paradigm and contributed significantly to solving health puzzles.

Integrative medicine

This paradigm shift in medicine was clearly signalled with the establishment of its own journal in 1998 called *Integrative Medicine: Integrating Conventional and Alternative Medicine*. In its first publication, the editor notes 'Paradigm shifts do not come easily in medicine' (Weil 1998). The extent of the paradigm shift can also be evidenced by the reason for the demise of the journal. With mainstream medical journals such as the *Journal of the American Medical Association*, the *New England Journal of Medicine* and the *British Medical Journal* requesting submissions in CAM and Integrative Medicine, and publishing works in these areas, the need for a separate journal was obviated.

In the USA, integrative medicine is being developed in an *ad hoc* manner and there is an increasing body of literature on individual experiments in creating integrative centres (Blanchet 1998). By 1998, it was reported that at least a dozen major medical schools had created programmes in integrative medicine. Most of these have occurred within schools of medicine while a number have brought together several schools such as nursing, medicine, social welfare, dentistry, and health technology and management. Such efforts face problems (Girard-Couture 1998) but are probably facilitated where there is a commitment to have outcome assessments of CAM as an integral part of the programme (Coulter 1999a). In the UK, the discussion and development has been stimulated by an initiative of the Prince of Wales, establishing a steering committee and working groups to examine the issue of integrative healthcare (Coates and Jobst 1998). In this initiative, rigorous research of both CAM and conventional healthcare is seen as the basis for integration. Within the UK the group was able to identify numerous examples of where CAM and conventional healthcare are provided alongside each other. Twenty-two such cases were surveyed and key components for success were identified. The study concludes that CAM will thrive in mainstream healthcare where it satisfies an unmet need but, for that to be successfully integrated, it will need to address four key issues: attitudes of both CAM and conventional providers; evidence of effectiveness and safety; ensuring adequate training; and funding.

The problems of meaning

The first, and perhaps the major, problem is what is meant by integrative medicine. Yet there have been few attempts to 'problematise' the concept. To begin with, there are two different terms used to describe the same phenomenon: 'integrated medicine' and 'integrative medicine' (Rees and Weil 2001). Unfortunately, in the USA, the concept integrated medicine may be easily confused with the notions of integrated medical systems (system integration), an area of increasing focus. However, most publications in the USA take integrative medicine to mean 'practicing medicine in a way that selectively incorporates elements of complementary and alternative medicine into comprehensive treatment plans alongside solidly orthodox methods of diagnosis and treatment' (Faass 2001: 119). It would seem that integrative medicine is seen as an end point, while integrating CAM is the process by which it is achieved.

Such a definition begs a fundamental question: what is the distinction between CAM and integrative medicine? For most of the experiments on integrative medicine described in the literature, what is involved is the adding of CAM to largely hospital-based medical programmes (Sol and Faass 2001) although some based on primary care practices have also been described (Rolfe and Hohenstein 2001). In these models, two different processes are occurring. One is that allopathic medical doctors are adding CAM therapies to their own training (acupuncture being a favoured one). In addition, there are Western-trained doctors also trained in other medical systems who are beginning to practise both approaches in the hospital setting (these are usually dually licensed individuals, but they are clearly seen as allopathic physicians).

The second approach is to bring CAM providers into conventional health centres (the more popular CAMs for this style of integration would appear to be chiropractic, naturopathy, non-medical acupuncture and massage therapists (Weeks 2001)). Another increasingly integrated group is holistic nursing; this includes spiritual healing and touch therapy. The involvement of these nurses is not new but the type of practice often is. In some models, the nurse practitioner is proposed as the hub of the organisation, coordinating the biomedicine (with its medical director) and the natural medicine (also with its own director, such as a naturopath).

Kailin (2001: 45) has noted that such attempts reveal a 'tangled web of tacit and explicit power relations'. He identifies four conceptual maps of integrative medicine carried by the key stakeholders, which need to be addressed if integration is to be achieved. The first is isolated integration patterns, where CAM is included but is held at arms length from biomedicine (that is, where there is not a close working relationship). Second, dominating integration patterns occur where 'integrative medicine is seen as an errant subset of biomedicine' (Kailin 2001: 46). CAM providers have very restricted roles and their function is to treat biomedically defined diseases with biomedical diagnoses. The third conceptual map is physician–provider patterns, where the medical physicians provide the CAM therapy and the CAM providers are marginalised. The fourth conceptual map he terms the transformative integration pattern, where CAM and biomedicine are seen in a dynamic relationship. Here collaboration is based 'on mutual respect, humility, and a spirit of inquiry in the context of close, collegial working relationships' (Kailin 2001: 46).

While no recent work has charted the prevalence of these various approaches, the National Center for Complementary and Alternative Medicine (NCAM) has issued a request for proposals to study the barriers to integrative medicine, in a tacit recognition that many of the programmes have not been successful. The most ardent supporters of integrative medicine espouse more than simply adding CAM to biomedicine. Indeed, Bell *et al.* (2002: 134) suggest that, in true integration, the incorporation of CAM would transform biomedicine. They state: 'As it evolves, truly integrative medicine also depends for its philosophical foundation and patient-centered approach on systems of CAM that emphasize healing the person as a whole (for example, traditional Chinese medicine, Ayuverdic medicine, and classic homeopathy)'. This is the same hope as that expressed in a recent *British Medical Journal* article (Rees and Weil 2001) which highlighted the beneficial effect of CAM on biomedicine. In their article, Rees and Weil (2001: 119) defined this form of integrative medicine as '[viewing] patients as whole people with minds and spirits as well as bodies and includ[ing] these dimensions into diagnosis and treatment'. There is a sense amongst some commentators that integrative medicine could be a unifying force in biomedicine (Reilly 2001). The editorial accompanying these two articles waxed even more philosophical: 'It mightn't be too pretentious (although it might) to say that such a growth might restore the soul to medicine' (Smith 2001). For some writers, integrative medicine is a way of bringing medicine back to its roots (Snyderman and Weil 2002) and, in this approach, allopathic physicians are not only educated about CAM and its benefits but also to adopt the basic patient–doctor paradigm thought to be characteristic of CAM practice.

There is, however, another approach to integrative medicine emerging within the CAM community itself, the insurance industry and with those termed by one writer as the CAM entrepreneurs (Weeks 2001). In areas such as chiropractic, networks have been formed both by health plans and by chiropractors themselves to begin 'integrating' their care in the delivery systems (Hanks 2001). In the case of chiropractic, articles are now appearing in the literature describing 'pursuing integration' (Simpson 2001). This type of integration may have financial benefits for the chiropractors (particularly in getting plan coverage) but also may greatly expand the resources they can get access to (X-Ray facilities, scans, laboratory tests, etc.). They may also gain access to other CAM providers, such as naturopaths, homeopaths, and practitioners of traditional Chinese medicine and of Ayuverdic medicine. The degree of integration may vary considerably, but in some programmes it does include clinical integration. But again, we have a range of meanings for integrative medicine from simply being part of a health plan and covered by insurance to integrating with medical care (Mootz and Bielinski 2001).

Last, but not least, another form of integrative medicine is that created by the patients themselves. In one sense, this was the first group to achieve integrative medicine. The increasing evidence about the use of CAM services (Trachtman 1994) shows that patients develop their own personal strategies for obtaining integrative care (Simpson 2001). In one sense, CAM providers and allopathic physicians are always connected in a network through their patients, even if this was never acknowledged. Few CAM providers are used exclusively by their patients. In the case of chiropractic patients, over 80 per cent of the patients retain the services of a medical physician (Kelner *et al.* 1980) and a more recent study (Eisenberg *et al.* 1998) suggests 83 per cent of patients who seek CAM treatment for serious medical conditions also consult a mainstream provider. To a large extent, it is the patient who determines when to use either an allopathic or CAM physician and how these are to be integrated into their health plan.

In conclusion, we can see from the above discussion that integrative medicine has many meanings and describes a whole range of social systems. Clearly, it has something to do with including CAM in orthodox medical practice (or the reverse). But even this is becoming problematic. While common definitions have defined CAM in terms of exclusion from medical schools, increasingly CAM is being included in medical school curriculums. Second, CAM covers a wide range of practices and belief systems that have very little in common with each other. The integration can be virtual integration or real bricks-and-mortar integration (Simpson 2001). It can be simply an administrative integration, a practitioner–system integration where the providers are linked economically and share facilities and services, or clinical integration where the services are coordinated across the patients.

The problems of integration

Perhaps the major problem confronting integrative medicine is finding a principle for integration. For some programmes the reason for integration has been simply financial. The data on use of CAM, and the data on the sums of money being spent on CAM by patients, convinced many that integration could be a money-making proposition. Shuval (2001) notes a similar motivation for hospital clinics in Israel. The evidence to date, however, is that few of the integrative medicine clinics are prospering financially (Hanks 2001). Many of the hospital-based programmes saw the inclusion of CAM as a way of retaining their client base and of filling beds. Eisenberg's study convinced many that one-third of their patients were using CAM (Coulter 1999a). Unfortunately for their hopes, most of CAM is focused on ambulatory care and maintaining patient mobility, and thereby keeps patients out of hospital.

A second major reason for integration was the fact that CAM users were often not informing their medical physician about such use. This meant that there was a real risk to the health of the patient from possible drug interactions. Surveys indicate that patients would welcome being able to discuss their CAM use with a physician who was knowledgeable about such medicines (Gaudet and Faass 2001). The principle here therefore was to improve the quality of the care delivered by increasing the comprehensiveness of that care.

However, whatever the reason, the challenge was to find a principle for the integration. One widely proposed principle was to integrate those CAM therapies for which there was evidence for efficacy. There is an increasing call within medicine for subjecting CAM to the same rules of evidence that are assumed to be held for medicine (Lewith and Aldridge 1993; Vickers 1996; Levin *et al.* 1997; Vickers *et al.* 1997; Chalmers 1998), and for the same methods of evaluation, such as assessment of clinical skills, and safety evaluations (Lewith and Davies 1966; Kingston 1996; Ernst and Barnes 1998). Astin *et al.* (1998) note that there are three major physician objections to CAM. The first is that CAM providers lack extensive knowledge, particularly with regard to diagnosis. A second is that there is a lack of evidence for efficacy. A third is that there is a risk for patients because they delay appropriate medical care by using CAM. A more radical position is that there is only one kind of medicine – that which has empirical support – and that until CAM can demonstrate this support it should not be considered complementary or alternative (Angell and Kassirer 1998). Richardson (2001) has described a project in a National Health Service (NHS) Hospital Trust to introduce CAM in the context of an evaluation programme. Lacking randomised controlled trials on which to base their selection of CAM, the Trust opted for a consensus conference to identify possible services and indicators for referral (using guidelines), the services (osteopathy, acupuncture and homeopathy), and evaluation of the services.

The position that evidence-based practice is the basis for integrating CAM and conventional medicine is fraught with difficulties and assumes that modern medicine is itself evidence based (see Willis and White, Chapter 3). Large parts of medicine could not meet such a strict criterion (Dalen 1998). Furthermore, such an approach implies that a standard of research which has taken conventional medicine close to a century to achieve (dating from the Flexner Report in 1910), should be met by the CAM group. The latter has had no research funding from National Institutes of Health (NIH) or the National Research Council until very recently, it is for the most part not located in the university system, and is practised in isolated, solo practices by individuals not trained as researchers. To expect CAM to compete on a level playing field with conventional medicine in research is unrealistic.

In its more extreme form, this position argues that science is the only basis for practice. This assumes that the practice of medicine has already been established as scientific. It has been suggested that CAM should be subjected to the same process, and some doubt whether CAM could survive the process (Federspil and Vettor 2000). Fontanarosa and Lundberg (1998: 1618) note 'There is no alternative medicine. There is only scientifically proven, evidence-based medicine supported by solid data or unproven medicine, for which scientific evidence is lacking.'

For many supporters of integrative medicine, the approach is simply to take those CAM therapies that have passed rigorous scrutiny and incorporate them into conventional medicine. But CAM is more than simply a set of therapeutic interventions. They are interventions that are given within a distinct health encounter and within, usually, a distinct philosophy of health and healthcare, both of which may have a direct and indirect impact on the efficacy, and more certainly the effectiveness, of such interventions. They form part of a distinct paradigm.

To claim that CAM must become evidence-based, however, is to make an epistemological claim, a preference for one form of knowledge over another. It is also a claim for the primacy of the epistemological basis of orthodox medicine. As Tonelli and Callahan (2001) note, this amounts to a philosophical demand. It involves two claims: that evidence-based medicine has provided a clear (and superior) value to orthodox medicine; and that it is applicable to all the healing arts. They note, even within orthodox medicine, there are other forms of knowledge that are equally compelling and may be more compelling. Also, 'medical epistemology cannot be separated from medical metaphysics' (Tonelli and Callahan 2001: 1214). So, while an epidemiologic epistemology may make sense within a biophysical theory of disease, it may not fit with other theories of disease. In CAM, both the individuality of the patient and the provider are thought to be key elements in the healing. But the methods most favoured in evidence-based practice, blinding, randomisation, placebos/control groups, for Tonelli and Callahan (2001) obscure these effects. Furthermore, care in CAM is seldom homogeneous. It is based on individualised care. Such heterogeneity makes it virtually impossible to do standard RCTs.

The question therefore is more rightly whether two quite distinct paradigms, biomedicine and CAM, having quite distinct philosophical foundations, distinct a priori assumptions and distinct metaphysical beliefs, can be unified within a single paradigm without doing great violence to at least one of the paradigms or totally transforming the other. This is a much more fundamental question than simply: Can medicine incorporate (co-opt) the best therapies of CAM into its therapeutic armamentarium? To understand this, we examine briefly the nature of these two paradigms.

Integrating paradigms

It is clear that integrative medicine is philosophically problematic. Not only are the paradigms of CAM and biomedicine incommensurable and non-comparable in the sense Kuhn outlined, but they may be built around contradictory metaphysics. In physics, either Newton or Einstein is right, but they cannot both be right. Time and space can either be absolute or relative but it cannot be both at the same time. In physics, the way this problem has been solved is that for the most part, and therefore for most phenomena, Newton can be treated as though his theory is correct even though we know, because of Einstein, that strictly speaking it is not. For most practical purposes, it is near enough. In those circumstances where it is not 'near enough' we switch to Einstein's theory. In this case, we do not actually solve the contradiction (time and space are absolute versus time and space are relative) but simply agree to tolerate it. There has been a lively debate in the philosophy of science about whether paradigms are totally incommensurable (Lakatos 1970).

The biomedical paradigm of health

In examining these two paradigms it is interesting to note that many of the CAM group, at least those from Western society (for example, homeopathy, naturopathy, osteopathy and chiropractic), arose out of a reaction to medicine in the latter part of the nineteenth century. Medicine, largely through the germ theory of disease, had begun its transformation from an art to a science. The germ theory of disease gave medicine its first spectacular success with so-called killer diseases. But, more significantly, it brought together the practice of medicine and the scientific method of investigation. Increasingly, medicine came to be less a purely clinical matter.

But this move toward science had distinct consequences for medicine. It involved a reductionist approach to illness. The search was for external, microscopic causes of disease in the first instance. Illness was reduced to disease, to disturbed pathology. It also elevated the concept of biological determinism. Causes of illness were looked for internally in the biological structure of the patient (Davidoff 1998). Health came to be seen as an absence of disease and the latter was explained in materialistic terms.

As a consequence, medicine came to be highly dependent on science. Medical arts became medical science, and medical schools either housed strong science departments within them or were highly integrated with science faculties. Medicine also came to be practised in different settings: those of the hospital and frequently those of the teaching hospital. Here, education and service have to compete with a mission that included the advancement of science through research. These tend to be large, bureaucratic and impersonal institutions. Diagnosis became complex and highly dependent on technology located in these same institutions, and frequently carried out by non-medical personnel. The twentieth century saw the demise of the solo general practitioner, the rise of the specialist and virtually the disappearance of care rendered at home.

The focus also changed, with acute illness and trauma taking precedence over chronic illness. The success of medicine has been much more extensive for the former two than for the latter. Nor has it been all that successful with the illnesses related to lifestyle. The very success of the germ theory of disease has also highlighted the limitations of medicine. Furthermore, the therapies of medicine became more radical with a concurrent increase in iatrogenic illness. Powerful therapies turned out, for the most part, to have powerful side-effects. In a perverse way, the focus on killer diseases also meant a focus on irreversible pathologies and the successes also highlight the failures.

The germ theory of disease therefore introduced a philosophical and therapeutic paradigm that transformed the notion of health, transformed the nature of medical practice, transformed the settings in which it was practised, and moved to a focus on the biological structure and disease as opposed to the individual and illness. This did not occur without some costs to human relationships and, in particular, to the doctor–patient relationship. It should be noted that many writers have seen this as a paradigm in crisis (Engel 1977, 1982; Pellegrino 1979; McWhinney 1986).

The CAM paradigm of health

While the CAM sector is extremely diverse, as noted earlier, many of the CAM group arose, or at least developed, in reaction to the medical paradigm and in particular to the germ theory of disease. Although this objection took many forms, it was seldom an outright rejection of the theory but more a recognition of its limitations, the most serious of these being the inability to account for the distribution of disease. Most of CAM postulates that the origin of disease, or health, comes not simply from external causes but from within the body. When disease occurs, it does so because of predisposing factors in the individual. Germs, under this approach, may be the initiating factor but lowered resistance is the predisposing factor. Biomedicine in this view attacks the effects or symptoms of disease but not the cause. The body, when functioning properly, is able to successfully combat disease, and illness is a failure in the body's natural restorative power. So germs by themselves do not cause disease.

This fundamental a priori difference leads to a different logic vis-à-vis treatment. In CAM, the focus is on treating the patient whose body will initiate the healing. The intention of the CAM practitioner is to assist the patient to heal him or herself. In this approach, diseases are symptoms of a more fundamental underlying cause. While the CAM group is very diverse and has varied meanings even amongst those who use them (Low 2001), there are some philosophical/metaphysical elements which most share (Coulter 1991). While writers have tried to isolate the major metaphysical elements shared by CAM, the extent to which they share them will vary. Also, different writers have identified different elements. Dovey (2001) identifies what he terms six naturopathic principles present in alternative medicine. These include: the healing power of nature; treat the whole person; first do no harm; identify and treat the cause not the symptoms; prevention is the best cure; the physician is a teacher. Eskinazi (1998) concludes that what these principles share are beliefs about vital force, spirituality and holism. In terms of spirituality, he notes many include beliefs from the cultures in which they develop: hence, traditional Chinese medicine is likely to include Taoist beliefs, Ayurvedic medicine a Hindu worldview and Tibetan meditation will include Buddhist concepts. Fulder (1998) chooses six basic health views which he feels characterise alternative medicine: self-healing is thought to be paramount; they work with, not against symptoms; they stress individuality, with each person's condition being different; individuals are regarded holistically and health involves the integration of human facets; illness has no fixed beginning or end; remedies conform to universal principles such as yin/yang. There is however considerable overlap in these various attempts to characterise CAM. So, while on the one hand we can accept that the CAM group represents a heterogeneity of practices (Tovey and Adams 1999), at a general level there are two distinct 'parent medical worlds represented by conventional medicine and CAM. Furthermore, we might begin our analysis by acknowledging that these worlds involve different (and sometimes opposing) views about the nature of diagnosis, illness and treatment' (Tovey and Adams 1999: 114). Here I identify the broad metaphysical positions that lie behind these philosophical principles.

Vitalism

Vitalism accepts that all living organisms are sustained by a vital force that is both different from, and greater than, physical and chemical forces. In the extreme form, the vital force is supernatural. A less extreme form is simply *vis medicatrix naturae* (the healing power of nature). Vitalism stands in direct opposition to materialism, which holds that disease can be explained entirely in terms of materialistic factors and therefore there is no need to invoke vitalistic forces. In philosophy, vitalism is usually held to be a metaphysical belief that failed the death of a thousand qualifications (Kekes 1973). Since materialism was held to explain everything, involving vitalistic forces was seen as unnecessary. In CAM there are numerous ways of expressing this Vitalism (*Qi,* life force, yin/yang, *prana*, universal intelligence, innate, etc.).

Holism

Holism postulates that health is related to the balanced integration of the individual in all aspects and levels of being: body, mind and spirit, including interpersonal relationships and our relationships to the whole of nature and our physical environment. Holism therefore is contradictory to the notion of reductionism since it holds that the whole is different from, and greater than, the sum of the parts.

Naturalism

Most of the CAM groups express a preference for natural remedies. This is bound up with a set of philosophical principles which may be expressed as: the body is built on nature's order; it has natural ability to heal itself; that this is therefore reinforced by the use of natural remedies; that it should not be tampered with unnecessarily through the use of drugs or surgery; and that we should look to nature for the cure. While we may debate the extent to which many of the substances of CAM are actually natural, there is this widespread acceptance of things natural.

Humanism

Humanism is based on the postulate that individuals have immutable rights, for example, the right to dignity. In CAM, there is extensive concern about the dehumanising procedures and the dehumanising institutions that have been created to care for the ill. Partly, it is recognition of the personal, social and spiritual aspects of health and is a move away from simply the biology of health. There is also a concern about the dehumanising nature of medical technology. Virtually without exception, CAM has been practised in small, solo practices where the dignity of the patient is considered an important part of the therapy.

Therapeutic conservatism

Most of CAM is therapeutically conservative: that is, it uses therapies that have a low level of side-effects and it tends to accept that the least care is the best care. This in some ways is derived from the earlier principle of vitalism. If the body is capable of healing itself, the role of the therapy is simply to initiate the process. Since continued care may intervene with this process, the intent is for minimal treatment. This is not to suggest that CAM treatment may not be extensive but only that philosophically it tends to be conservative. Much of CAM care is oriented to getting the patients to be active on their own behalf and reducing therapeutic dependency.

Out of these metaphysical principles, we can derive a particular philosophy of health and a particular philosophy of healthcare.

Philosophy of health

In CAM, health is the natural state and the innate tendency of the body is to restore health. Health is also the expression of biological, socio-psychological and spiritual factors, and optimal health is unique to an individual.

Philosophy of healthcare

In terms of healthcare, CAM makes several major distinctions. First, it distinguishes between disease and illness. In this approach, disease is seen as dis-ease, or a body that has a lack of ease. Second, it distinguishes between health and disease. Health is not simply the absence of disease but involves a patient achieving their full potential in light of their biological, psychosocial and spiritual limitations. Third, CAM distinguishes between treatment and care. The objective of CAM is to care for the whole person, not simply treat the symptoms. Fourth, health involves optimising homeostasis in the body. Health is seen as holistic and therefore involves optimising holistic responses. Fifth, the practitioner is seen as merely a facilitator and an educator. Health is not seen as something given by the provider to the patient (health comes from within or not at all). It is seen as an achievement of the patient and the provider both facilitating the body's innate ability to heal.

Again, while the CAM group is diverse, members do share a similar view on the nature of health and healing. Montgomery (1993) has argued that the apparent heterogeneity among the CAM group hides a unity that derives from a few fundamental premises. For him, these are located around the discourse on holism. His own analyses of the discourse concludes 'one discovers that the language employed, particularly with regard to discussing disease directly, tends to form a closed system erected upon a distinct range of central terms and images' (Montgomery 1993: 71).

Integration of the two paradigms

As outlined above, in many ways biomedicine and CAM begin with what seem like incompatible, if not contradictory, fundamental assumptions. Cassidy (1995) notes that each group examines illness from different paradigms that reflect two different ways of constructing reality in our society. One is that used by bioscientists (reductionism) and one is used by alternative healthcare (holism). 'Listening to such conversations, one has the impression that unbeknownst to the speakers, two languages are being spoken' (Cassidy 1995: 20). To an anthropologist or sociologist, this should come as no surprise since both disciplines subscribe to a theory about the social construction of realities and the primacy of the worldviews that arise from these constructions.

One possible scenario for trying to integrate CAM into medicine is that the therapies of CAM will be adopted (co-opted) by medicine (or at least, the successful ones) without the philosophical elements. A second scenario might be termed the Trojan horse scenario, that is, CAM will be integrated and this will transform the nature of medicine surreptitiously. The question here is whether the therapies alone will have the same success when they are stripped of the paradigm within which they traditionally resided. It may be the case that these approaches are effective because they are incorporated in a broad-based 'wellness' paradigm. A third option is to formulate a meta-paradigm that will allow for these two to coexist.

Systems theory

The most likely candidate for formulating such a metaparadigm is a systems theory approach. Systems theory has been seen as a conceptual way of integrating and organising knowledge within and across disciplines, from physical and biological sciences to the behavioural and social sciences (Schwartz and Russek 1997). Systems theory emerged in modern physics to solve the problem that the characteristics of individual parts of a system change according to their context (Ranjan 1998). So the study of parts is insufficient without a study of their relationships and the changing contexts. The same element can differ in changing contexts and the focus is on organisational complexity. As noted by Dacher (1995), the biomedical model is based on the assumptions of objectivism, determinism and positivism. The alternative model incorporates three aspects of being: instinctual, mind/body and spiritual. He proposes a model that can incorporate biomedicine that has three principles: dynamism, holism and purposefulness. The model is based on systems theory. Dacher proposes a hierarchy of healing systems that provide the link between cellular physiology and social adaptability. In the initial triage, the objective is to identify not simply the symptoms but the healing system to be applied. The systems of healing he identifies are: 1) the homeostatic healing system, which is a built-in instinctual physiologic system that automatically responds to internal states of disequilibrium; 2) the treatment healing system, which involves a healthcare practitioner (but which he sees as unable to include psychological, psychosocial and spiritual factors); 3) the mind/body healing system, such as psychoneuroimmunology and which includes psychological and psychosocial factors; and, 4) the spiritual healing system. These four systems of healing are considered an integrated comprehensive system. In treating a patient, the provider must decide which of the systems is to be applied to the present problem.

Beckman *et al.* (1996) have similarly proposed a systems model of healthcare. They see the advantage of systems theory as being that it approaches both biological and psychological systems within a holistic context. Systems theory, as applied to living organisms, embraces several characteristics that make it an ideal candidate for integrating CAM and traditional medicine. These include the conceptualisation of the body as a multilevelled structure that has a set of interrelated and mutually dependent organisational levels of differing complexity. Systems theory also has an ecological view of the relationship between the organism and its environment. Changes in the environment, or the individual, will synchronously affect each other. Systems theory posits the notion of interactivity and a non-linear causality. There is a process of mutually interactive and self-reinforcing feedback that both maintains and transforms a system. Systems theory also recognises the principle of self-organisation. There is an inherent capacity to return to a balanced state (homeostasis). In addition, living systems have the capacity to transcend any one state and create new structures and forms of organisation that are unpredictable. In systems theory, the mind is a manifestation of the same set of systemic properties as life itself. Mind represents the dynamics of self-organisation. The mind as the organising process is inherent in all systems and at all levels of life.

A further element in systems theory is the concept of emergent properties (Bell *et al.* 2002). Not only is the whole greater than the sum of its parts but the larger systems have properties that are simply not found in the parts or in their summation.

The most favoured candidate for systems theory in the health field is that formulated initially by Engel as the biopsychosocial model (Engel 1977, 1980). As Schwartz and Wiggins (1986) note, if the biopsychosocial model is to be framed as a systems theory, it must use concepts that can be applied to all systems – biological, psychological and social. The strength of Engel's model, they feel, is the recognition that health and illness occur in the inter-connections of these systems. The systems are both independent of each other but also dependent on them. One of the functions of systems is to reduce complexity. At the biological level, this is done through our organs so that, for example, in the eye, rods and cones select some inputs and negate others. At the psychological level, meanings perform a similar function. For Schwartz and Wiggins (1986), our biology selects things in a vague and global way, but a suprabiological structure (meanings) has evolved to supplement the biological ones. Such meanings are developed through our own individual development but also through socialisation, in which we take up the perspectives of others. Meaning structures therefore impose constraints that supplement biological structures, and both reduce complexity for the individual and establish a correspondence between the psychological and social systems, therefore regulating interactions between these systems.

For an increasing number of authors, it is within CAM that we find the fullest expression of Engel's model. Bausell and Berman (2002) go so far as to suggest that the increasing popularity of CAM may be due to the fact that this is where the public is encountering this model and are not finding it in biomedicine or psychiatry (the field for which Engel proposed it). CAM patients do seem to be attracted to providers who claim to treat the whole person. Siahpush (1998) has shown that postmodern values of the population (those about nature, science, technology, health, authority, individual responsibility and consumerism) are the most predictive of attitudes towards alternative therapies. For Bausell and Berman (2002), the move to CAM by the public changes the framework in which medicine is viewed. 'What we are observing is really nothing less than a genuine Kuhnian paradigmatic shift in world views' and, further, it 'may represent a consumer-driven variant of George Engel's call for an actual reformulation of what is meant by the practice of medicine itself' (Bausell and Berman 2002: 31).

This also brings us full circle because it challenges the notion that integrative medicine is simply biomedicine with CAM added.

> Combination medicine (CAM added to conventional) is not integrative. Integrative medicine represents a higher order system of care that emphasizes wellness and healing of the entire person (bio-psycho-socio-spiritual dimension) as primary goals, drawing on both conventional and CAM approaches in the context of a supportive and effective physician–patient relationship.
>
> (Bell *et al.* 2002: 133)

While the authors also state that integrative medicine is not CAM, they do suggest that 'as it evolves, truly integrative medicine also depends on its philosophical foundations and patient-centered approach on systems of

CAM that emphasize healing the person as a whole' (Bell *et al.* 2002: 134). Employing systems theory, we can identify in integrative medicine those emergent properties not found in any of the component parts. It has also been suggested that CAM practitioners have maintained a philosophy of health that increasingly resonates both with public demand and the health needs of the public (Coulter 1999b). It is at the level of philosophy that the CAM systems really are distinct from biomedicine and are truly alternative.

Conclusion

CAM presents an interesting challenge for medicine. On the one hand, medicine has to acknowledge that despite its massive opposition to, and denigration of CAM, these medicines are growing in popularity. From 1997 to 1998, the growth in reported inclusion of CAM in Health Maintenance Organisations (HMOs) in the USA grew from 43 per cent to 67 per cent. About 48 per cent of HMO members report having access to alternative care (Landmark Healthcare Inc. 1999). The dilemma for medicine is whether to embrace alternative medicine or to become increasingly removed from a major part of their patients' healthcare.

As documented, there is evidence that many institutions are opting for a move to integrative medicine as a way of combating the challenge posed by CAM. This will pose a serious intellectual challenge as two historically antagonistic, sometimes contradictory and frequently contrary paradigms, are brought together. In the area of system theory, there is the opportunity for an integrative theory that has gained considerable acceptance in the biological sciences and medicine and which can incorporate many of the principles of alternative healthcare. The history of medicine has shown an extraordinary ability to convert yesterday's heresy into today's healthcare. At the same time however, the incorporation may lead to a transformation of the biomedical paradigm. The Trojan horse may turn out to be the apt metaphor.

References

Agassi, J. (1964) 'The nature of scientific problems and their roots in metaphysics' in Bunge, M. (ed.), *The Critical Approach to Science and Philosophy*, London: Free Press, pp. 189–211.

Angell, M. and Kassirer, J.P. (1998) 'Alternative medicine – the risks of untested and unregulated remedies', *New England Journal of Medicine* 339,12: 839–41.

Astin, J.A., Marie, A., Pelletier, K.R., Hansen, E. and Haskell, W.L. (1998) 'A review of the incorporation of complementary and alternative medicine by mainstream physicians', *Archives of Internal Medicine* 158,21: 2303–10.

Bausell, R.B. and Berman, B.M. (2002) 'Commentary: alternative medicine. Is it a reflection of the continued emergence of the biopsychosocial paradigm?', *American Journal of Medical Quality* 17,1: 28–32.

Beckman, J.F., Fernandez, C.E. and Coulter, I.D. (1996) 'A systems model of healthcare: a proposal', *Journal of Manipulative and Physiological Therapeutics* 19,3: 208–15.

Bell, I.R., Caspi, O., Schwartz, G.E., Grant, K.L., Gaudet, T.W., Rychener, D., Maizes, V. and Weil, A. (2002) 'Integrative medicine and systemic outcomes research: issues in the emergence of a new model for primary healthcare', *Archives of Internal Medicine* 162,2: 133–40.

Blanchet, K.D. (1998) 'University Center for Complementary and Alternative Medicine at Stony Brook', *Journal of Alternative Complementary Therapies* 4,3: 327–32.

Cassidy, C.M. (1995) 'Social science theory and methods in the study of alternative and complementary medicine', *Journal of Alternative Complementary Medicine* 1,1: 19–40.

Chalmers, I. (1998) 'Evidence of the effects of healthcare: A plea for a single standard across 'Orthodox' and 'Complementary' medicine', *Complementary Therapies in Medicine* 6: 211–13.

Coates, J.R. and Jobst, K.A. (1998) 'Integrated healthcare: a way forward for the next five years? A discussion document from the Prince of Wales's Initiative on Integrated Medicine', *Journal of Alternative Complementary Medicine* 4,2: 209–47.

Coulter, I.D. (1991) 'An institutional philosophy of chiropractic', *Chiropractic Journal of Australia* 21: 136–41.

Coulter, A.H. (1999a) 'The new Cedars-Sinai Alternative Medicine Clinic. Expansion of healthcare for the community', *Journal of Alternative Complementary Therapies* 5,2: 93–8.

Coulter, I.D. (1999b) *Chiropractic. A Philosophy for Alternative Health Care*, Oxford: Butterworth-Heinemann.

Dacher, E.S. (1995) 'A systems theory approach to an expanded medical model: a challenge for biomedicine', *Journal of Alternative Complementary Medicine* 1,2: 187–96.

Dalen, J.E. (1998) '"Conventional" and "unconventional" medicine: can they be integrated?', *Archives of Internal Medicine* 158,20: 2179–81.

Davidoff, F. (1998) 'Weighing the alternatives: lessons from the paradoxes of alternative medicine', *Ann Intern Med* 129, 12: 1068–1070.

Dovey, D. (2001) 'Basic principles of complementary/alternative medicine', *Clinicians Complete Guide to Complementary/Alternative Medicine*, St Louis: Moseby, pp. 5–7.

Eisenberg, D.M., Davis, R.B., Ettner, S.L., Appel, S., Wilkey, S., Van Rompay, M. and Kessler, R.C. (1998) 'Trends in alternative medicine use in the United states, 1990–1997: results of a follow-up national survey', *Journal of the American Medical Association* 280,18: 1569–75.

Engel, G.L. (1977) 'The need for a new medical model: a challenge for biomedicine', *Science* 196,4286: 129–36.

Engel, G.L. (1980) 'The clinical application of the biopsychosocial model', *American Journal of Psychiatry* 137,5: 535–44.

Engel, G.L. (1982) 'Sounding board. The biopsychosocial model and medical education. Who are to be the teachers?', *New England Journal of Medicine* 306,13: 802–5.

Ernst, E. and Barnes, J. (1998) 'Methodological approaches to investigating the safety of complementary medicine', *Complementary Therapies in Medicine* 6: 115–21.

Eskinazi, D.P. (1998) 'Factors that shape alternative medicine', *Journal of the American Medical Association* 280,18: 1621–3.

Faass, N. (2001) *Integrating Complementary Medicine into Health Systems*, Gaithersburg: Aspen Publishers.

Federspil, G. and Vettor, R. (2000) 'Can scientific medicine incorporate alternative medicine?', *Journal of Alternative Complementary Medicine* 6,3: 241–4.

Fontanarosa, P.B. and Lundberg, G.D. (1998) 'Alternative medicine meets science', *Journal of the American Medical Association* 280,18: 1618–19.

Fulder, S. (1998) 'The basic concepts of alternative medicine and their impact on our views of health', *Journal of Alternative Complementary Medicine* 4,2: 147–58.

Gaudet, T.W. and Faass, N. (2001) 'Developing an integrative medicine programme: The University of Arizona Experience' in Faass, N. (ed.), *Integrating Complementary Medicine into Health Systems*, Gaithersburg: Aspen Publishers, pp. 35–40.

Girard-Couture, C. (1998) 'Integrating natural medicines into allopathic hospital pharmacies', *Journal of Alternative Complementary Therapies* 4,3: 249–51.

Hanks, J.W. (2001) 'Chiropractric inclusion in complementary and alternative medicine clinics: Analysis of current trends', *Topics in Clinical Chiropractic* 8,2: 20–25.

Kailin, D.C. (2001) 'Initial strategies' in Faass, N. (ed.), *Integrating Complementary Medicine into Health Systems*, Gaithersburg: Aspen Publishers, pp. 44–58.

Kekes, J. (1973) 'The rationality of metaphysics', *Metaphilosophy* 4: 124–39.

Kelner, M., Hall, O. and Coulter, I.D. (1980) *Chiropractors, Do They Help*, Fitzhenry and Toronto: Whitesides.

Kingston, S. (1996) 'The assessment of clinical skills for practitioners of complementary medicine', *Complementary Therapies in Medicine* 4: 202–3.

Kuhn, T. (1962) *The Structure of Scientific Revolutions*, Chicago: University of Chicago Press.

Lakatos, I. (1970a) 'Falsification and methodology of scientific research programmes' in Musgrave, A. (ed.) *Criticism and the Growth of Knowledge*, London: Cambridge University Press, pp. 91–196.

Landmark Healthcare Inc. (1999) *Landmark Report II. HMOs and Alternative Therapy*, Sacramento.

Levin, J.S., Glass, T.A., Kushi, L.H., Schuck, J.R., Steele, L. and Jonas, W.B. (1997) 'Quantitative methods in research on complementary and alternative medicine. A methodological manifesto. NIH Office of Alternative Medicine', *Medical Care* 35,11: 1079–94.

Lewith, G. and Aldridge, D. (1993) *Clinical Research for Complementary Therapies*, London: Hodder and Stoughton.

Lewith, G. and Davies, P. (1966) 'Complementary medicine: the need for audit', *Complementary Therapies in Medicine* 4: 233–6.

Low, J. (2001) 'Alternative, complementary or concurrent healthcare? A critical analysis of the use of the concept of complementary therapy', *Complementary Therapies in Medicine* 9,2: 105–10.

McWhinney, I.R. (1986) 'Are we on the brink of a major transformation of clinical method?', *Cmaj* 135,8: 873–8.

Montgomery, S.L. (1993) 'Illness and image in holistic discourse: how alternative is "alternative"', *Cultural Critique* Fall: 65–89.

Mootz, R.D. and Bielinski, L.L. (2001) 'Issues, barriers, and solutions regarding integration of CAM and conventional healthcare', *Topics in Clinical Chiropractic* 8,2: 26–32.

Pellegrino, E.D. (1979) 'Philosophical groundings for treating the patient as a person: a commentary on Alisdair MacIntyre' in Siegler, M. (ed.) *Changing Values in Medicine*, New York: University Publishers of America, pp. 99–103.

Ranjan (1998) 'Magic or logic: Can "alternative" medicine be scientifically integrated into modern medical practice?', *Advances in Mind–Body Medicine* 14: 43–73.

Rees, L. and Weil, A. (2001) 'Integrated medicine', *British Medical Journal* 322,7279: 119–20.

Reilly, D. (2001) 'Enhancing human healing', *British Medical Journal* 322,7279: 120–1.

Richardson, J. (2001) 'Developing and evaluating complementary therapy services: Part 1. Establishing service provision through the use of evidence and consensus development', *Journal of Alternative & Complementary Medicine* 7,3: 253–60.

Rolfe, L.K. and Hohenstein, K.A. (2001) 'Strategic planning in the integration of complementary medicine' in Faass, N. (ed.) *Integrating Complementary Medicine into Health Systems* Gaithersburg: Aspen Publishers, pp. 76–89.

Schwartz, G.E. and Russek, L.G. (1997) 'Dynamical energy systems and modern physics: fostering the science and spirit of complementary and alternative medicine', *Alternative Therapies in Health Medicine* 3,3: 46–56.

Schwartz, M.A. and Wiggins, O.P. (1986) 'Systems and the structuring of meaning: contributions to a biopsychosocial medicine', *American Journal of Psychiatry* 143,10: 1213–21.

Shuval, J.T. (2001) 'Collaborative relationship of alternative practitioners and physicians in Israel', *Complementary Health Practice Review* 7,2: 111–25.

Siahpush, M. (1998) 'Postmodern values, dissatisfaction with conventional medicine and popularity of alternative therapies', *Journal of Sociology* 34,1: 58–70.

Simpson, C.A. (2001) 'Pursuing integration: a model of integrated delivery of complementary and alternative medicine', *Topics in Clinical Chiropractic* 8,2: 1–8.

Smith, R. (2001) 'Restoring the soul of medicine' (Editorial), *British Medical Journal* 322: 117.

Snyderman, R. and Weil, A.T. (2002) 'Integrative medicine: bringing medicine back to its roots', *Archives of Internal Medicine* 162,4: 395–7.

Sol, N. and Faass, N. (2001) 'Integrative medicine programs in hospital environments' in Faass, N. (ed.), *Integrating Complementary Medicine into Health Systems*, Gaithersburg: Aspen Publishers, pp. 90–5.

Tonelli, M.R. and Callahan, T.C. (2001) 'Why alternative medicine cannot be evidence-based', *Academic Medicine* 76,12: 1213–20.

Tovey, P. and Adams, J. (1999) 'Thinking sociologically about complementary medicine', *Complementary Therapies in Medicine* 7,2: 113–15.

Trachtman, P. (1994) 'NIH looks at the implausible and the inexplicable', *Smithsonian* 25: 110–23.

Vickers, A. (1996) 'Methodological issues in complementary and alternative medicine research: a personal reflection on 10 years of debate in the United Kingdom', *Journal of Alternative Complementary Medicine* 2,4: 515–24.

Vickers, A., Cassileth, B., Ernst, E., Fisher, P., Goldman, P., Jonas, W., Kang, S.K., Lewith, G., Schulz, K. and Silagy, C. (1997) 'How should we research unconventional therapies? A panel report from the Conference on Complementary and Alternative Medicine Research Methodology, National Institutes of Health', *International Journal of Technology Assessment in Health Care* 13,1: 111–21.

Wartofsky, M.W. (1967) 'Metaphysics as a heuristic for science' in Wartofsky, M.W. (ed.), *Boston Studies in the Philosophy of Science III*, Reidel Publishing Company: Dordrecht, pp. 123–72.

Watkins, J.W.N. (1958) 'Confirmable and influential metaphysics', *Mind* LXVII: 344–65.

Weeks, J. (2001) 'Major trends in the integration of complementary and alternative medicine' in Faass, N. (ed.), *Integrating Complementary Medicine into Health Systems*, Gaithersburg: Aspen Publishers, pp. 4–11.

Weil, A. (1998) 'Editorial', *Integrative Medicine* 1,1: 1.

Chapter 7

CAM practitioners and the professionalisation process

A Canadian comparative case study

Heather Boon, Sandy Welsh, Merrijoy Kelner and Beverley Wellman

Introduction

Attempts by complementary and alternative medicine (CAM) practitioners to achieve professional status are not new. What may be new, however, is the increasing number of different CAM practitioner groups seeking legitimate status as healthcare practitioners throughout the industrialised world. For example, in the province of Ontario, Canada, naturopathic practitioners, traditional Chinese medical practitioners, acupuncturists and homeopathic practitioners are all striving for professional status codified in state-sanctioned regulation (Wellman *et al.* 2001). In Britain, both osteopathic and chiropractic practitioners have recently been regulated, and the House of Lords Report recommends regulation for acupuncture and herbal medicine (Select Committee on Science and Technology 2000). And in the USA, chiropractors, naturopathic practitioners and acupuncturists are being regulated in an increasing number of states. The professionalisation of CAM practitioner groups appears to be a widespread phenomenon, yet relatively little is known about how these practitioner groups are making the transition from occupation to profession.

The difficulties of defining the term 'profession' and the myriad definitions that have been proposed led Freidson to suggest that researchers clarify what they mean when discussing professions and the professionalisation process (Freidson 1983). For the purposes of our analysis, we are defining the gaining of statutory self-regulation or state-sanctioned professionalisation as being equivalent to the professionalisation process. The three CAM occupations we explore in this chapter are focused on the goal of state-sanctioned regulation and are at various stages in reaching it. Much of the discussion of professionalisation in the practitioner focus groups described in this chapter concentrated on what would happen when they gained this legal status, what the barriers were to achieving this status, and who their allies and competitors were in the pursuit of it. Statutory self-regulation was a central theme in all our focus groups.

Much of the research in the area of professionalisation focuses on conflicts over jurisdictional claims, quests for state-sanctioned self-regulation,
and attempts at social closure. The vast majority of studies of professionalisation explore the pure professions (medical doctors and lawyers) and the
professionalisation attempts of female-dominated 'semi' professions such
as nurses and midwives. Since the 1990s, researchers of CAM have increasingly used professionalisation theories to understand what is happening
with CAM practitioners (Saks 1995; Cant and Sharma 1996). We build on
these studies by examining the relevance of two important concepts in the
study of professions: social closure (Collins 1990; Saks 1995) and jurisdictional boundaries (Abbott 1988). Although social closure has received
a fair amount of attention in recent analyses of CAM, Abbott's work on
jurisdictional boundaries and the system of professions has been less
prominent.

We take as the starting point for our case study the views of practitioners
from three CAM groups in Ontario, Canada: naturopathic practitioners,
homeopaths and traditional Chinese medicine/acupuncture practitioners. By
focusing on the experiences of the practitioners themselves, we move away
from a focus on what the leaders of the CAM associations say they are
doing and the 'party line' that often supports these strategies. What our
analysis offers is an examination of the challenges CAM practitioners
believe they face as their group strives for statutory self-regulation.

The professionalisation process

Researchers who study the professionalisation process have a range of
theories to choose from when seeking to explain the strategies employed
by various occupational groups. One well-known approach, trait theory,
looks at specific characteristics needed by an occupation to professionalise.
Another approach to examining CAM occupations may be to incorporate
issues of power, monopoly and complex interactions within CAM groups,
between CAM groups, as well as between CAM groups and the other
medical professions. To gain a better understanding of the latter approach,
we utilise two perspectives from the study of professions: social closure
(for example Collins 1990) and the system of professions (Abbott 1988).

Social closure explains part of the success some groups have had in working toward professional status. This concept

> refers to the process by which occupational groups are able to regulate
> market conditions in their favour in face of competition from outsiders
> by limiting access to a restricted group of eligibles, enabling them effec-
> tively to monopolize available opportunities.
>
> (Saks 1998: 176)

Certain healthcare groups, such as medicine and dentistry, have been masters at social closure. They have been able to exclude others from gaining jurisdictional control or statutory self-regulation. For modern professions, statutory self-regulation or state licensure is a primary way to achieve market closure. Whether the CAM occupations in our analysis will attain state-sanctioned regulated status is an important part of our question.[1]

The concept of social closure helps us to understand part of the picture of the professionalisation of CAM groups. But, as noted by others, social closure approaches do not fully account for the interactions amongst professional groups nor for processes other than exclusion in determining who gains control (Adams 1998). This is where the work of Andrew Abbott may be helpful for rounding out our understanding of the professionalisation of CAM groups.

Abbott's work highlights how professions are organised into a system, and he argues that it is more useful to analyse this system rather than analyse individual professions in isolation (Abbott 1988). A system approach regards the jurisdictional claims professions make as they assert their authority and/or try to gain status as being linked to the claims of other groups in the system. Abbott discusses the social, structural and cultural dimensions of jurisdictional claims made by professions. Professions may ask for 'absolute monopoly of practice and of public payments, rights of self discipline and of unconstrained employment, control of professional training, of recruitment, and of licensing, to mention only a few' (Abbott 1988: 59).

Claims may be made to the media, the legal system or the political system. For Abbott, it is not the content of the claims that is important, but the location, form and 'the social structure of the claiming professions themselves' (Abbot 1998: 59) that is of most interest. Abbott also argues that, as opposed to the trait approach to professions, 'a profession is not prevented from founding a national association because another has one. It can create schools, journals, and ethics codes at will. But it cannot occupy a jurisdiction without either finding it vacant or fighting for it' (Abbott 1988: 86). Following this reasoning, we see that the conventional medical establishment cannot stop the CAM occupations from organising and founding their own schools and associations. But it is the contests over jurisdiction, that is, where CAM practitioner groups will find space for their claims, that ultimately will determine the relative success of the various CAM professionalisation projects (Abbott 1988).

Abbott also notes that legally determined jurisdictions for professions tend to rigidly define what it is the profession does. He states 'Boundary areas are firmly delineated with formal definitions that are in fact uninterpretable in actual situations' (Abbott 1988: 63–4). Herein lies, in part, the rationale for examining the views of practitioners about the professionalisation process. It is the practitioners, in the course of their actual work, that choose to work within (or outside) the boundaries as defined by their professional associations and/or government statutes. The ambiguities between how the practitioners view their work, as compared to the official goals of their practitioner group, constitute a key point for investigation of the professionalisation process.

Most studies of the professionalisation process have focused on the formal views of leaders. Here, we take a different approach, asking practitioners themselves about their work and their views concerning the professionalisation of their occupations and thereby examining the micro-level dimensions of professionalisation. Although we are looking at three distinct CAM occupations, and not necessarily the overlap between them, we see these occupations as making jurisdictional claims within much the same territory: first, the territory already claimed by mainstream medicine in general and, second, the territory of clients looking for alternatives (or complements) to mainstream medicine.

Case study: naturopaths, homeopaths and traditional Chinese medicine/acupuncture practitioners in Ontario, Canada

Methods

Three focus groups (one with practitioners from each occupation of interest) were held in Toronto, Ontario, Canada. Participants were randomly sampled from lists of practitioners obtained from the various practitioner associations. The lists were supplemented by names of practitioners obtained from other sources such as internet listings, advertisements in local health magazines and personal contacts. Every effort was made to ensure that the lists were complete before the sample was drawn. Selected practitioners were mailed or faxed a letter of introduction, followed by a telephone call from a team member to determine their availability and willingness to attend the focus group at the scheduled time. In addition, to meet the inclusion criteria, they were required to be eighteen years of age or older, be actively involved in treating patients a minimum of twenty hours per week and be able to communicate in English well enough to provide informed consent and participate in a group discussion.[2]

Each focus group was led by a moderator who guided the group through a series of topics for discussion. The moderator began by posing general and broad questions to each focus group including: 'Are you aware of any professionalisation or attempts to be regulated going on for your occupation?' 'Do you think professionalisation or regulation is a good idea? Why, or why not?' Additional probes were used as needed. Another investigator also attended each focus group in order to compare field notes and discuss the group process. Each two-hour session was audiotaped and transcribed verbatim.

The transcripts of each focus group were coded independently by four investigators using a constant comparative analysis (Berg 1989). The central issues that emerged in each group were identified through the key concepts or phrases used by participants during the discussion. After every focus group, the four investigators met to compare and combine their independent analyses. Such simultaneous data collection and analysis made it possible to explore and expand on themes from earlier focus groups at subsequent sessions. During the next phase of the analysis the investigators identified similarities, contrasts and potential connections among the concepts within and amongst each focus group. The final step in the analysis involved the development of the major themes and the identification of phrases or quotations that most accurately illustrated these themes. The software program QSR Nvivo (2001) was used to organise and code the data on the relevant themes.

Findings

The participants

The naturopathic focus group comprised five naturopathic practitioners, all educated at the same Naturopathic College in Toronto. Four out of the five were members of the same two naturopathic associations. The other individual did not list membership in any associations. Participants had been practising for an average of three and a half years. Four were women and three were born in Canada. The average age of the focus group participants was thirty-nine years. All participants were contacted as part of a random sample of naturopaths.

There were five participants in the traditional Chinese medicine (TCM)/ acupuncture focus group. Four received their training in China (one of these four also received conventional medical training from a Canadian medical school). The fifth participant received training in acupuncture from an association that provides acupuncture training to primarily Western-oriented medical doctors. Two participants were members of a Western-oriented acupuncture association, two were members of one of the Canadian TCM-based associations, and one was a member of a different Canadian TCM-based association. Participants had been practising TCM/ acupuncture for an average of twelve and a half years. Three participants were male and two were female. None of the participants were born in Canada, with four of them listing China as their country of origin. The average age of the participants was fifty-three years. Two of the participants were contacted as part of the random sample, while three were contacted through personal networks.

Ten homeopaths participated in the homeopathic focus group. Six were trained at the same college in Ontario, the other four were trained at different colleges, including one in the UK. Participants listed themselves as members of five different professional associations, with five of the ten informants belonging to the same Ontario homeopathic association. The participants reported being in practice for an average of five and a half years. Four participants were male and six were female. Four of the homeopaths were born in Canada; the other six were born in Eastern Europe, the UK or India. The average age of participants was forty-four years. Seven participants were contacted as part of the random sample while three were contacted through personal networks.

Key themes

Statutory self-regulation was clearly identified as the goal of the professionalisation process by the CAM practitioners in our focus groups. All the practitioners asserted that their CAM group was pursuing statutory self-regulation under the Regulated Health Professions Act (the Act under which all healthcare practitioners in Ontario are currently regulated). Most, but not all, personally felt this was an important goal for their occupational group. The other three key issues that emerged from the focus group discussions were: the struggle to effect social closure; the challenge of lack of cohesion and jurisdictional battles within the individual practitioner groups; and the question of whether their work should be considered a profession or a single-practice modality. These are discussed in detail below.

SOCIAL CLOSURE

A long list of reasons for seeking statutory regulation was identified in all the focus groups. Many of these related to the groups' attempts at social closure. For example, all three practitioner groups expressed the opinion that statutory regulation would result in some form of monopoly with respect to the therapies they practice:

> Homeopathy is also the stepchild of each and every profession in North America. If you are a chiropractor you practice homeopathy along with it. If you're a naturopath, homeopathy is used in your practice. If you are a massage therapist . . . if you are a midwife, you use homeopathy . . . and you can count not one, but twenty other areas . . . some kind of regulation will clear this area of various part-time professionals.
>
> (Homeopathy focus group)

> The impression I get is that if you're in the newer Act you have a little more security and, as well . . . have more of a monopoly which unfortu-

nately is the essence of the profession. That you need to be able to say, look I can do this and proportionally you can't and we have the legal whatever . . . recourse at our disposal to make sure that no one else can come in as a whatever . . . naturopathic impersonator and take over what we're doing because we've been trained under a certain statute or whatever.

(Naturopathy focus group)

The groups tended to see regulation as a means to prevent the co-optation of their skills and knowledge by other professional groups:

I think we have a window of opportunity to come together and try to pursue some sort of regulation because if we don't what's going to happen in the future is that some other profession will dilute homeopathy, perhaps medical doctors or specialists.

(Homeopathy focus group)

Unless you establish yourself with a college, with a piece of paper, what your stages are, who should enter the program, what the program is going to be, and who will regulate the program, then you only become a section of a recognized medical discipline.

(Acupuncture focus group)

But the thing is if we do get recognition in HPRAC [Health Professions Regulatory Advisory Council] then we can say look to the OMA [the Ontario Medical Association] . . . you know, you actually have restrictions. You cannot be practicing this stuff; this is our scope of practice. You do not have experience with whatever it may be and, you know, please desist or otherwise we'll have to take legal action. So, you can put some pressure on other groups that are doing what we do, whether it's homeopathy or whatever. So, I think it still would help us from my perspective.

(Naturopathy focus group)

Co-optation is the process by which one group embraces within their scope of practice techniques or treatments that were originally developed by or solely practised by another group. Physicians have been accused by many CAM groups of 'CAM-poaching' – incorporating the 'best' or 'scientifically proven' CAM treatments within the jurisdiction of medicine in a bid to eliminate the need for CAM practitioners. Co-optation was a real fear that was compounded by the real or perceived overlap between what each group claimed as their own jurisdiction or 'work'. Homeopaths, the least cohesive of the groups, appeared most worried about jurisdictional overlap with their fellow CAM practitioners, the naturopathic practitioners. For their part, naturopaths and TCM/acupuncture practitioners were most concerned about already regulated medical professions:

> I think with the naturopaths we're really not sure whether we should be paranoid or embrace them because we're not sure whether they will swallow us up or not.
>
> (Homeopathy focus group)

> Competitors? I personally see the regular professions practicing acupuncture as competitors, for example, massage therapists.
>
> (Acupuncture focus group)

Added to these general competition concerns were concerns about claiming jurisdiction based on judgments about who was best trained to provide specific types of CAM care:

> I tend to agree that MDs pose the greatest threat in the sense that they subsume a naturopathic approach, albeit in 5 minutes.
>
> (Naturopathy focus group)

> I mean the naturopaths study approximately 200 hours in the entire four years of homeopathy and then a lot of them use it as a namesake because it is the one connection in all the modalities.
>
> (Homeopathy focus group)

Most practitioners felt that regulation would allow them to achieve a measure of social closure by instituting education and qualification standards that would prevent others from practising on their turf:

> I think if it's regulated there will be certain restrictions and people won't be allowed to practice that don't have the proper background or they will have to re-educate.
>
> (Homeopathy focus group)

> . . . that [regulation] to me from my perspective is a good thing because it will ensure that the quality of education is maintained at a certain level and even improved . . .
>
> (Naturopathy focus group)

> We must have a set of regulations so everyone can meet the regulations, before they can practice.
>
> (Acupuncture focus group)

LACK OF COHESION AND INTERNAL JURISDICTIONAL BATTLES

One of the key challenges facing the groups' attempts at social closure is the lack of internal cohesion within the practitioner groups themselves:

> It's really important though that the community try to come together instead of breaking off into factions because we're not powerful to the government when we're all broken up into small groups. We need to come together as one large cohesive group and that's the only way. I mean I think the government likes it this way because it's easy to deal with us this way. It's much harder if we come together and are one large powerful group.
>
> (Homeopathy focus group)

> I don't understand why we're just so scattered . . . why we're not just a unifying strong group.
>
> (Naturopathy focus group)

Social closure strategies such as setting educational or practice standards can only be effective if the group can agree on the content and form of those standards. All the practitioner groups identified this as a challenge facing their group; however, it appears to be particularly problematic for the homeopaths and the TCM/acupuncture practitioners, who have a wide variety of training institutions and associations struggling for control of the profession in Ontario:

> What we haven't been able to do in 200 years is get along.
>
> (Homeopathy focus group)

> I think one of the barriers is the homeopathic community itself with their different opinions of regulation, as well as their different opinions on standards. . . . So, we can't actually agree on anything as a group.
>
> (Homeopathy focus group)

> How many nuclei have started, right? [laughter] That is the problem, right?
>
> (Acupuncture focus group)

Some of the fragmentation that is evident within the practitioner groups is a result of diverse practice styles and philosophies. Establishing standards is exceedingly difficult because the practitioners who are attempting to professionalise actually practise different forms of each modality. Emerging from the homeopathic and TCM/acupuncture focus groups was the need to determine who would 'win' the internal jurisdictional battles before statutory self-regulation could occur:

> I'm not speaking for anyone else in the room because I don't know any of these folks, but I have seen a lot of anger be directed at the kind of homeopathy that I include in my practice. It's not the only thing I do, but it is part of what I do and so there are some ways in which bringing the groups together can be very difficult and particularly people who feel strongly about regulation also tend, not always, but tend to feel strongly about the right way to practice. So, if you've got two groups who both feel strongly about the right way to practice, but the two groups don't agree, it means bringing them together is very difficult.
>
> (Homeopathy focus group)

> The only thing we have in common is the Law of Similars, that's it. Other than that, we practice differently. So, strong feelings are going to come because somebody is going to be accused of suppression or whatever else.
>
> (Homeopathy focus group)

> I see lots of conflicts in the group. One is standards: we don't want those who don't know acupuncture to practice acupuncture; we don't want those who don't know traditional Chinese Medicine to practice it . . .
>
> (Acupuncture focus group)

Some practitioners feared a loss of freedom to practise as they wished if their practitioner group was regulated:

> I agree with you to a certain extent, if you're saying the use of the Chinese model. But what about Korean acupuncture? In Korean acupuncture, the diagnosis is a bit different, so they have another mode of medicine. If they say acupuncture belongs to Chinese medicine only, that means you exclude other practitioners who practice other types of acupuncture.
>
> (Acupuncture focus group)

> I would say wonderful if that were the case, but history teaches us when you bring in regulation, you also bring in restriction and that's not reality, as much as we would all around this table like to say how nice that would be. I mean I fully agree with you, it would be wonderful if we could regulate and be completely open and we're only talking about minimum standards of education and some basic surrounding knowledge . . . it would be really nice to have that kind of surrounding

set of standards, but historically . . . I mean look at the massage therapists. Of all the schools, surely massage would be the most flexible, but if you're not Swedish massage, you're not an RMT.

(Registered massage therapist)

So, if you practice shiatsu and get 22:00 hours in training in anatomy and physiology and massage, you can not call yourself an RMT. So, the Swedish massage people are saying this is the only real way of doing massage and we know that's nonsense, but that's what is most likely to happen if we regulate.

(Homeopathy focus group)

PROFESSION VS. MODALITY

Another issue raised by both the homeopathic practitioners and the TCM/acupuncture practitioners was the confusion over whether the therapy they practised was a profession in its own right or was simply a modality that could be employed by a variety of healthcare professionals. Currently, homeopathy and acupuncture are seen as both professions and modalities, which makes regulation of these practices exceedingly challenging. For the TCM/acupuncture group this issue was particularly acute. The week before the focus group, the Health Professions Regulatory Advisory Council (HPRAC)[3] released their recommendations about the future regulation of TCM and acupuncture in Ontario. In their recommendations, the HPRAC stated that they will consider acupuncture a modality, not a profession (Health Professions Regulatory Advisory Council 2001b).

I am a bit confused about the whole situation. It sounds like there is a proposal that acupuncture is a treatment modality and that TCM is TCM. I don't know why we have to argue that acupuncture is a Chinese thing. Acupuncture, since 1973, has been known to the West, specially in North America and a lot of things have been developed since then. . . . To me, acupuncture is a form of physical therapy just like giving an injection. In traditional Chinese medicine, when you practice acupuncture, you also use injections of whatever substance, and there are schools in North America using similar techniques but they developed differently from different roots than acupuncture, so, I must say, that acupuncture treatment, I cannot agree with you that it belongs to Chinese medicine.

(Acupuncture focus group)

I agree that acupuncture can be viewed as a modality, but there is a line you have to draw. I can stretch this to an extreme . . . in the gynecology department, the nurse might use one needle to induce labour . . . so everyone can practice acupuncture because the applications are very high. However, for this you don't define acupuncture as a profession, but as a treatment of modality that can be used by a variety of professions. And as for regulation, it is just technique. . . . If the professionalisation of radiation therapist or radiologist are being proposed by this report, the analogy can be drawn that radiation therapy can be treated as a modality. It can be prescribed and utilised by a nurse, if they were only trained for, say, a month, for just one type of breast cancer, then to prescribe one particular drug. . . . This is the analogy. Is there anything wrong? To some patients there might not be anything wrong, but to the bottom line that it defines a profession as basically a territory of practice . . . why can't a person trained for thirty days prescribe something a little bit more than Tylenol? . . . It doesn't work that way because of the need of the professions.

(Acupuncture focus group)

This highlights the fact that the CAM practitioner groups are trying to carve out 'turf' in a healthcare system already overflowing with professions. They appear to realise that they need to find a place to 'fit' within the system (as opposed to the current situation where they operate outside the system):

I think that one of the goals of us as a profession is to be more integrated into the health consciousness of Ontario, Canada; to be integrated into the health system and part of that is looking professional in the eyes of conventional medicine and the peers in that field so that that transition runs smoothly . . . that they will accept us more readily if we have the qualifications, the professional demeanor and what not. I think that's another reason to head towards regulation, towards this process of professionalisation.

(Homeopathy focus group)

One of the biggest allies for all the CAM practitioner groups who are attempting to find their place within the healthcare system is the public:

I think that the one thing which is happening is the pressure from the public because there are more people who are seeking the naturopathic services and I think it has changed in the last five years. This is one group of informed public who is helpful to our profession.

(Naturopathy focus group)

Other allies are the communities of people. In Toronto we have communities of people whose first medicine is homeopathy and if it doesn't work, then it is allopathy. One of them is the Muslim community, they have a spiritual homeopath and they have a weekly session on TV on homeopathy. They provide a centre of service from England as to what to take on what health condition people send them. So that's one big group in and around Toronto. I don't know the number. Then you have an East Indian community. Many of them will use homeopathy first.

(Homeopathy focus group)

There is evidence that the groups feel a need to change (their rhetoric if not their practice) to fit into the current healthcare system. For example, the homeopaths (and the naturopathic practitioners) have recast their 'work' as possibly harmful (as opposed to the view previously popularised that CAM is perfectly safe). This is in response to the Ontario criterion requiring that a practice must have potential for harm before it is eligible to be regulated:[4]

I also know that there are a few obstacles, one of which that the prime directive of the college network in Ontario is you have to first prove you're dangerous, which is easier to do with acupuncture and naturopathy and chiropractic medicine than it is with homeopathy.

(Homeopathy focus group)

Discussion

Our data indicate that many of the key issues associated with the professionalisation of health occupations – the quest for state-sanctioned self-regulation, attempts at social closure and conflicts over jurisdictional claims – are clearly relevant for the professionalisation of CAM practitioner groups. Statutory self-regulation is the ultimate 'prize' coveted by all the practitioner groups, despite the fact that it may not be a goal for all individual practitioners. Overall, the groups expect that regulation will provide the necessary power to effect social closure around their 'turf'. However, their efforts to gain social closure are hampered by a variety of barriers, including lack of internal cohesion, battles of jurisdiction and the need to fit into a healthcare system with no obvious need for additional professions.

The fragmentation within each occupation – as is particularly evident for the homeopathic and TCM/acupuncture communities – appears to be the single biggest obstacle for the groups to effect social closure. However, another key obstacle is what Abbott would term the lack of 'vacancies' in the current system of professions (Abbott 1988). There are already twenty-four health professions regulated in the province of Ontario (O'Reilly 2000), and there are no obvious gaps waiting to be filled by CAM practitioners. It appears that CAM practitioners currently perform some of the 'dirty work' in the system by specialising in treating difficult or undesirable patients, such as those with elusive complaints that have not been helped by conventional care and those that are dissatisfied with the conventional system. In this way, CAM practitioners may be attempting to carve out a specific jurisdiction within the system and thus their patients may be their greatest allies when arguing the need for formal regulation.

The situation is complicated further by the social context of the regulated healthcare professions in Ontario, Canada. The legislative review process, begun in the 1980s and culminating in the 1991 Regulated Health Professions Act, had the goal of 'increasing the coordination and cooperation of the health professionals' (O'Reilly 2000: 199). The new Act includes a description of each regulated profession's scope of practice that provides 'information about what the profession does, the methods it uses, and the purpose for which it does these things' (O'Reilly 2000: 83), but is not meant to outline exclusive practice territories. Rather than licensing practitioners per se, the Act focuses on licensing specific acts or procedures that are deemed potentially harmful. These 'controlled' or 'authorised' acts can legally be performed only by specific professional groups authorised by the statute to perform them. Within this context, any attempts by CAM practitioner groups to effect social closure around a specific jurisdiction are made more difficult.

The situation has recently become even more challenging for the TCM/acupuncture community. The recommendation by HPRAC that acupuncture should be regulated as a modality, not a profession (Health Professions Regulatory Advisory Council 2001b), is problematic for gaining social closure and a full jurisdictional claim by one group that establishes their 'complete legally established control' (Saks 1998: 71). The report recommends that the government of Ontario establish a system of limited jurisdictional control of acupuncture for several professions, including doctors, nurses, TCM practitioners and physiotherapists.

This highlights the need for the CAM practitioner groups to find a way to 'fit' into the existing system of professions. The history of chiropractors in Ontario[5] suggests that CAM practitioner groups may need to accommodate their practice (and perhaps their philosophy of care) to fit into the conventional healthcare system if they hope to attain their stated goal of statutory regulation (Biggs 1989, 1994; Boon 1996). HPRAC has identified nine criteria by which they judge who should be given professional status in Ontario, and each CAM group must provide a submission to this Council providing a justification of how they meet each criterion. This context provides the rules by which the CAM groups must play. What is not clear is how conforming to these requirements will ultimately affect the scope of practice of the CAM practitioners (and the work that they do) if they ultimately become regulated healthcare practitioners in Ontario. How 'alternative' will they remain? Our data provide a useful baseline for future research of these issues.

Our results highlight key areas for further research. It is important to note that we collected data from a very small group of participants that is likely not to be representative of CAM practitioners in Ontario or elsewhere. The aim of this qualitative study was to explore the range of experiences of CAM practitioners who are members of different groups at different stages in the professionalisation process. While our findings are not conclusive, they do provide sensitising concepts and building blocks for theory generation. Only future studies with larger samples across a number of CAM occupations can assess the generalisability of our findings.

Conclusions

Writing about the situation in the UK, Saks states that '[e]ven the professionalisation of alternative medicine may not be as challenging as first meets the eye' (Saks 1998: 185). In Ontario, even though the CAM practitioner groups continue to experience significant internal fragmentation, HPRAC has recommended that both naturopathic medicine and TCM/acupuncture be regulated and has provided some direction on how this should be accomplished[6] (Health Professions Regulatory Advisory Council 2001a; Health Professions Regulatory Advisory Council 2001b). On the surface at least, the government is no longer standing in the way of the regulation of CAM practitioner groups. However, the HPRAC reports emphasise that the CAM groups are responsible for setting educational and practice standards and, given the current divisions within the groups (especially TCM/acupuncture), this could prove difficult. Clearly, achieving internal cohesion is one of the key challenges facing CAM groups attempting to professionalise. Another important challenge is whether CAM practitioners can maintain their distinct philosophies of care and unique practices within the regulatory framework to be imposed upon them. Additional research in this area will be critical in order to enhance our understanding of the professionalisation process.

The Ontario, Canada context for CAM professions shows both the usefulness and limits of the social closure perspective. Some degree of social closure will occur when the goal of statutory self-regulation is achieved, but it will not create a monopoly for some of the therapies that the CAM groups practise, acupuncture in particular. Due to the way regulation is structured in Ontario, other medical professions will still have the right to include some types of CAM work in their practices. This is where an analysis that includes the complex system of professions is needed – in particular, where more attention to the work of Andrew Abbott may shed light on the continuing jurisdictional battles between CAM groups and between CAM and conventional medicine. Abbott's emphasis on how boundaries between professions are established at the workplace site, or through the work practitioners do, may prove helpful for understanding the system of CAM and conventional medical professions (Abbott 1988). This is especially relevant, as CAM becomes more integrated in the health-care system, hospitals and multi-disciplinary medical clinics throughout the world.

The professionalisation of CAM groups is necessarily constrained by the healthcare and regulatory systems in which it is occurring; however, the key components of the process are likely to be similar. Studies comparing the professionalisation of CAM practitioners in different countries would greatly enhance our knowledge of this process. In addition, longitudinal studies investigating the professionalisation project over time will provide insight, especially with respect to assessing the extent to which CAM prac-titioner groups compromise their distinct identities for state-sanctioned legitimacy. This chapter makes a strong case that all future studies in this area must investigate the professionalisation of CAM within the context of the system of professions.

Notes

1 Self-regulatory status, with some degree of social closure, does not guarantee cultural legitimacy: chiropractors are a good example of this. In other work, we examine the relationship between statutory self-regulation and cultural legitimacy. Because of the stress placed on statutory self-regulation by the practitioners in our focus group, we focus on that.
2 The exclusion of non-English speakers may have had a bearing on our results, especially for the TCM/acupuncture group. This warrants further investigation.
3 The Health Professions Regulatory Advisory Council (HPRAC) has a mandate to review issues related to the Regulated Health Professions Act (including requests from new occupations wishing to be regulated under the Act) that are referred to it by the Minister of Health, and to make recommendations to the Minister (O'Reilly 2000).
4 The nine criteria used to determine who should be given professional status in Ontario are: (1) Relevance of the proposed self-regulating group to the Ministry of Health; (2) Risk of harm to the public; (3) Sufficiency of supervision; (4) Alternative regulatory mechanisms; (5) Body of knowledge; (6) Education requirements for entry to practice; (7) Ability to favour pubic interest; (8) Likeli-hood of compliance; and (9) Sufficiency of membership size and willingness to contribute (O'Reilly 2000).
5 Chiropractors significantly narrowed their scope of practice during their bid for state-sanctioned self-regulation. This strategy, which was successful for them, is detailed in several recent dissertations, for example, Boon (1996: 290) and Biggs (1989).
6 Homeopathy has not yet been formally referred for review by HPRAC by the Minister of Health and Long-term Care.

References

Abbott, A. (1988) *The System of Professions. An essay on the division of expert labor*, Chicago: University of Chicago Press.

Adams, P. (1998) 'Drug interactions that matter. (1) Mechanisms and management', *The Pharmaceutical Journal* 261: 618–21.

Berg, B. (1989) *Qualitative Research Methods for the Social Sciences*, Toronto: Allyn and Bacon.

Biggs, C.L. (1989) 'No Bones About Chiropractic? The quest for legitimacy by the Ontario Chiropractic Profession, 1895–1985', PhD Dissertation in Department of Behavioural Science/Community Health, Toronto: University of Toronto.

Biggs, C.L. (1994) 'The silent partner? The state's role in the formation of the Ontario chiropractic profession's identity 1925–52', *Health and Canadian Society* 2: 35–62.

Boon, H. (1996) 'Canadian Naturopathic Practitioners: The Effects of Holistic and Scientific World Views on Their Socialization Experiences and Practice Patterns', PhD Dissertation In Faculty of Pharmacy, Toronto: University of Toronto.

Cant, S. and Sharma, U. (1996) 'Demarcation and transformation within homeopathic knowledge: a strategy of professionalization', *Social Science and Medicine* 42: 579–88.

Collins, R. (1990) 'Market closure and the conflict theory of professions', in Burrage, M. and Torstendahl, R. (eds) *Professions in Theory and History: Rethinking the Study of the Professions*, London: Sage.

Freidson, E. (1983) 'The reorganization of the professions by regulation', *Law and Human Behaviour* 7: 279–90.

Health Professions Regulatory Advisory Council (2001a) *Advice to the Minister of Health and Long-Term Care, Naturopathy*, Toronto.

Health Professions Regulatory Advisory Council (2001b) *Traditional Chinese Medicine and Acupuncture, Advice to the Minister of Health and Long Term Care*, Toronto.

O'Reilly, P. (2000) *Health Care Practitioners. An Ontario case study in policy making*, Toronto: University of Toronto Press.

Saks, M. (1995) *Professions and the Public Interest. Medical power, altruism and alternative medicine*, London: Routledge.

Saks, M. (1998) 'Professionalism and health care', in Field, D. and Taylor, S. (eds) *Sociological Perspectives on Health, Illness and Healthcare*, Oxford: Blackwell Science, pp. 176–91.

Select Committee on Science and Technology (2000) *Complementary and Alternative Medicine*, London: House of Lords.

Wellman, B., Kelner, M.J., Boon, H. and Welsh, S. (2001) 'Complementary and alternative leaders address the professionalization process', *Alternative Therapies in Health and Medicine* 7: S36.

Chapter 8

Demarcating the medical/ non-medical border

Occupational boundary-work within GPs' accounts of their integrative practice

Jon Adams

Introduction

Amidst the recent movement towards integrated healthcare, a small yet growing number of general practitioners (GPs) are personally practising complementary and alternative medicines (CAM). Based on transcripts from twenty-five in-depth interviews conducted with GP therapists, this chapter critically examines doctors' explanations and presentations of their integrative practice. Focus is placed upon a specific area of occupational boundary-work identified within the GPs' accounts: namely, the non-medical/medical divide. The exploratory study situates the doctors' boundary-work amidst the ongoing debates between different healthcare providers regarding the authentic location and ownership of CAM.

General practice and CAM

Alongside the more general expansion of CAM (Ernst 2000; MacLennan *et al.* 2002) has emerged a climate increasingly sympathetic to healthcare pluralism and integration (Featherstone and Forsyth 1997) with a growing interest in CAM from across the health and social care professions (Rankin-Box 1997; Henderson 2000; Adams and Tovey 2001). Studies have identified increasing interest in, referral to, and practice of CAM by primary care physicians in a number of countries including Australia (Easthope *et al.* 2000; Hall and Giles-Corti 2000; Pirotta *et al.* 2000), the USA (Berman *et al.* 1998; Grant *et al.* 2000) and Israel (Sarel *et al.* 1998; Vinker *et al.* 2002). This chapter focuses upon similar trends evident in the context of general practice in the UK (Perry and Dowrick 2000).

The British Royal College of General Practitioners has shown an interest in CAM (Honigsbaum 1985) and a number of grass-roots models of integration have been evolving within this branch of UK medicine (Adams and Tovey 2000). In particular, several studies have identified a small yet growing number of general practitioners who are personally practising one or a range of CAM in addition to more conventional medicines to treat their NHS patients (Perkin *et al.* 1994; Thomas *et al.* 1995; Botting and Cook 2000; Lewith *et al.* 2001; Thomas *et al.* 2001; Schmidt *et al.* 2002). Such a style of integration – direct integrative practice (Adams and Tovey 2000) – is the focus of this chapter.

The sociology of integrative practice

Some sociological research has begun to focus attention upon the integration of CAM within the medical profession (Saks 1995). Saks has examined the recent change in approach of the medical profession towards CAM – from outright criticism and ridicule to tolerance and consideration of the therapies for practice. Saks suggests integration should be understood primarily as a defensive strategy serving the self-interest of the medical profession and particularly the medical elite (Saks 1995).

Notwithstanding the merits of Saks' analysis, this past work has placed particular attention upon the stance of the medical elite towards CAM incorporation, examining formal documents and journal articles. The fact that the grass-roots of the medical community constitute a key site of enthusiasm about integrative practice (Nicholls 1988) (which has often been out of tune with the stance of the medical elite (Sharma 1992)) supports a reorientation of research focus upon the accounts of GPs personally practising CAM within their NHS surgeries.

More recent study has already begun such a reorientation of focus upon the grass-roots of the profession. May and Sirur (1998) have investigated a number of issues of concern to GP homeopaths, and Dew (2000) has explored the approach of practitioners, alongside that of others in general practice, to CAM in New Zealand.

While maintaining the focus upon GP therapists' accounts, this chapter also offers an original approach to the analysis of CAM integration within general practice. This work provides a specific focus upon occupational boundary-construction and introduces a conceptual framework underdeveloped in the sociology of CAM. Before detailing the study and its findings, the conceptual framework utilised is outlined.

A focus upon GP accounts and boundary-work

> When the goal is *expansion* of authority or expertise into domains claimed by other professions or occupations, boundary-work heightens the contrast between rivals in ways flattering to the ideologists' side.
>
> (Gieryn 1983: 791–2)

This research builds primarily upon key features from Gieryn's boundary-studies approach (also known as the cultural cartographic approach) developed from and utilised within science studies (Gieryn 1983, 1995, 1999). Gieryn himself has suggested that boundary-studies may be appropriate for the investigation of physicians and the medical profession (Gieryn 1983: 792). Recent work has employed this approach to examine collaborative healthcare practice (Allen 2000), the division of health labour (Allen 2001; Norris 2001) and the field of new genetics (Kerr *et al.* 1997). However, such studies remain notable exceptions in the literature and a boundary-studies approach is both still underdeveloped with regard to the sociology of health and illness generally, and absent from the growing examination of CAM and its changing relationship with the medical profession more specifically.

The boundary-studies perspective is primarily constructivist in that it conceives of the terrain and boundaries of a profession not as predetermined or fixed but as the outcome of ongoing negotiation and struggle within the profession and beyond (Gieryn 1995). Adopting this theoretical framework produces a fresh analysis of the medical/non-medical boundary, acknowledging the work of grass-roots doctors in producing and reproducing both the territory of their professional community and also the borders between them and other groups of practitioners. In tune with calls for a grass-roots perspective upon the direct integration of CAM within general practice (Adams and Tovey 2000), the demarcation of what can be legitimately classified as medicine from that which is classified as non-medicine is to be examined as 'a practical problem for [doctors]' (Gieryn 1983: 781).

In relation to GPs and CAM, 'boundary-work' here refers to the professional ideological efforts within doctor therapists' accounts both to distinguish their work from that of a whole host of other healthcare professionals and to maintain and enhance their authority and dominance in the healthcare arena. While Gieryn focuses upon the 'public sphere', there is equal validity to the study of accounts in a less public setting – in this case GPs' accounts produced through interview.

A boundary-studies approach shares a commonality with discursive and rhetorical psychology in that it critiques traditional interpretations of informants' accounts. Rhetorical psychology suggests that talk should not be treated simply as descriptions mirroring reality, but should be seen as inherently performative and persuasive (Billig 1991; Potter 1996). All explanations are constructed at the expense of alternative tellings and in this sense all talk can be said to be ideological in that it privileges a particular interpretation of the world over that of others (McInlay and Potter 1987).

However, while discursive psychologists and related writers restrict themselves to examining the *locale* of talk production (Potter 1996), this research aims to move beyond such an analysis to provide an examination of how informants' talk is inextricably linked to the wider social and political context. This approach seeks to help reintroduce the 'inferential nerve'

(Halfpenny 1988) to the analysis of informants' accounts, as outlined in earlier boundary-studies research (Kerr *et al.* 1997).

GPs demarcate boundaries and territory in everyday work sites, conferences, public speeches and other settings which involve dealings with GP colleagues, nurses, health service managers, secretarial staff and patients amongst others. This study sets out to analyse GP therapists' accounts of integrative practice (and the occupational demarcations therein) with a view to current professional struggles over the practice and location of resources relating to CAM.

Various routes are available for producing such an analysis of accounts (Kerr *et al.* 1997; Allen 2000). These include: ethnographic study of real work sites (Allen 2001); examining the pronouncements and debates found in the press, professional journals and conferences (Gieryn 1995); and interviews with key stakeholders (Norris 2001). In line with previous boundary-studies work (Kerr *et al.* 1997; Norris 2001), this research draws upon interview data collected from informants. The study explores the rhetorical strategies employed by GP therapists to establish and maintain occupational boundaries between themselves and non-medical therapists. This chapter does not report *real* differences between the two groups of practitioners, but outlines how individual practitioners (GP therapists) express occupational differences in their talk.

Method

This exploratory study comprised twenty-five in-depth unstructured interviews conducted with GPs practising CAM in the cities of Edinburgh and Glasgow, Scotland. Ten of the interviewees were practising acupuncture, sixteen practising homeopathy, twelve practising hypnotherapy and four neurolinguistic programming (some doctors were practising more than one therapy). The therapies included in the study were not chosen by the researcher. Instead, the inclusion criteria for the study were those therapies practised by the GPs who completed interviews. However, it is interesting to note that acupuncture, homeopathy and hypnotherapy – three therapies which have been shown to be well represented in wider samples of GPs (Thomas *et al.* 1995) – are also well represented amongst the twenty-five GPs recruited for the study.

All twenty-five GPs interviewed were in group practices of three or more partners. All apart from three had been practising for more than five years and twenty for over ten years. The interviewees comprised fourteen male and eleven female GPs. Interviews ranged from just under one hour to two hours in length and often varied owing to the time constraints upon the individual practitioners. Interviews were conducted at the GPs' health practices (often in between or immediately following normal consulting hours), either in their consulting room or another quiet vacant room nearby.

Assurances of confidentiality were given and the interviews audio-taped with the doctors' consent. At the close of the interview field notes were recorded as a means of documenting the overall experience of the interview session. All tapes were transcribed to computer files shortly following interview and transcription occurred concurrently with data collection and preliminary analysis throughout the fieldwork period.

The conceptual framework guiding the study does not emphasise the 'micro' details of talk, such as repetitions, extended pauses and overlappings often associated with discourse analysis and related perspectives. Instead, building upon the broad approach of Gieryn's boundary-studies (Gieryn 1983) and its utilisation in previous work (Kerr *et al.* 1997; Allen 2000), the research concentrates on registering the general claims and arguments used by the GPs to demarcate themselves from others and on contextualising such boundary-work in terms of occupational competition over the practice of CAM.

The study employed in-depth interviews; as far as possible, prompts were used only to ask for clarification or expansion of an informant's points. The interviews did not follow a formal interview schedule. Instead, key themes, arguments and words as mentioned by the GP were noted as the interview commenced and then consulted to further probe the GP's arguments and claims at a later stage in the interview.

Codes and analytical themes were developed in a cumulative manner in relation to particular claims and arguments identified from the GPs' accounts. In order to enhance the reliability of the analysis, an independent examination of sections of the interview transcripts was undertaken by two additional qualitative social science researchers. These additional researchers were given selected samples of transcripts from ten of the completed interviews (these passages were selected for independent analysis because they were deemed problematic in terms of interpreting codes and analytic themes). Issues regarding the coding of the data were then discussed by all three researchers (including the author) and any comments or suggestions fed back into the coding process. Internal validity was also considered to ensure the rigour of the study. Following the creation of coding files and preliminary analysis, the data were re-examined for evidence of negative cases of which none were identified.

Demarcating a medical/non-medical boundary

A specific area of occupational boundary-work identified within the GPs' accounts relates to a non-medical therapy/GP therapy divide. The doctors employ a number of different rhetorical devices with which to distance themselves and their practice of unconventional therapies from that of the non-medically qualified. This boundary-work hinges upon a presentation of contrasting styles of CAM practice.

Complementary as opposed to alternative: perceptions of styles of practice

> I'm an allopathic doctor. I use it as a complementary therapy rather than as an alternative. I'm not a homeopath I'm an allopath who uses homeopathy . . . alternative replaces, complementary is an add on.
>
> (GP 2)

> I've always considered these therapies complementary in the sense of being additive to orthodox medicine.
>
> (GP 18)

There has been much discussion and debate regarding a suitable and appropriate nomenclature for the therapies and medicines currently practised predominantly outwith the medical profession. Concern has been raised over the wider connotations of different labels; however, these have until now been mainly academic wrangles (Sharma 1992). Nevertheless, different labels and their respective connotations are also powerful discursive tools which can be deployed by different groups and their members who are actively involved and enmeshed in the arena of healthcare itself (Vickers 1993; Joyce 1994; Atkinson 1996; Botting and Cook 2000). The analysis presented here illustrates the role of different terminology and titles in the occupational boundary-work of 'rank and file' doctors.

Effectively, the doctors in the study perceive their style of therapy and practice as *complementary*, while in contrast they understand lay therapists to be involved in *alternative* therapy and likewise to be *alternative* practitioners. The GPs construe these two styles as fundamentally opposed and therefore as mutually exclusive in practice. As one GP therapist practising acupuncture, homeopathy and hypnotherapy explains:

> If it's complementary then they have to take on board what other allopractic medicine is offering and be willing to work along with that, and if you are then it's complementary. If they believe allopractic medicine is negative and is destructive and shouldn't ever be entered into then they're alternative . . . I'm complementary in that I would utilise these things as part of my armamentarium.
>
> (GP 15)

These banners of alternative and complementary practice are forcefully employed by the GPs to mark a non-medical therapy/general practice divide. The model of alternative therapy acts as a powerful rhetorical construction with which non-medical therapy is characterised as deficient and potentially highly dangerous.

The centrality of a conventional diagnosis and a conventional medical context

At the heart of the alternative-complementary divide and the GPs' attack upon non-medical therapy is a description of the importance of the conventional diagnosis. Some GPs explain how they see their practice and role as built primarily upon being a diagnostician. To quote a GP acupuncturist:

> My first job of all as a Western doctor is to diagnose and say yes I think this is a tension headache, there are a number of alternative treatments for you or I don't think this is a tension headache I think we should be investigating this more deeply and organising CAT scans. Perhaps my main job, my first job is diagnosis and *that's the most important thing I do*.
>
> (GP 24)

While many of the GPs note that there are alternative diagnostic systems associated with certain unconventional medicines (for example, in the case of acupuncture and homeopathy), these are often used to contrast a GP approach to the therapies with the approach of the non-medically qualified. One GP acupuncturist explains:

> I suppose in the process of diagnosis it's very much Western medicine. I mean if a patient comes to me with let's say neuralgia or an inflamed joint I would use Western medicine including if necessary blood tests and X-rays to make the diagnosis. I wouldn't, as a traditional Chinese healer would, use appearance of the tongue or twenty-one different pulses to try and determine a diagnosis, in terms of yin yang imbalance, you know I wouldn't. My diagnosis is very much based on erm traditional Western scientific principles.
>
> (GP 18)

Images of the scientific approach of conventional medicine, with particular reference to diagnostic procedures, pervade much of the GPs' boundary-construction between non-medical and general medical practice. The rhetoric of science is employed to underpin and contextualise the therapies and to distance GP practice from that of the non-medically qualified. An interviewee exemplifies the 'work' of this rhetoric of science regarding the GP's diagnosis and its necessity alongside unconventional therapy when she states:

> I think *science* gives you confidence [with complementary therapy]. I think if you look at somebody and think this person's for example hyperthyroid and you check the thyroid function and you *scientifically*

confirm this then obviously you can bang on in there and treat it with great confidence. If you couldn't check the bloods you would be treating it expectantly and hopefully and seeing if there was a clinical improvement so yeah the *scientific* side of it is important. It's important for the confidence of both people that you've got the right diagnosis.

(GP 3)

In this quote, scientific checks and confirmation, at least as a basis to certain medical practices, are presented as enhancing the utility and effectiveness of unconventional therapy. When analysed in these terms, we can see how the notion of *complementary* practice is one which implies the domestication of unconventional therapies within a wider framework of conventional scientific medicine. *Complementary therapy*, as constructed in the accounts of these GPs, implies a fundamental limitation to unconventional practice – a limitation which is perceived by these conventional doctors as more restrictive than non-medically qualified practitioners acknowledge or promote.

Contrasting rhetorics of safety and risk

[Lay therapists] are not approaching it from the medical point of view and it's kind of the safety first attitude really.

(GP 9)

The GPs' talk of diagnostic skills also links to their use of the contrasting rhetorics of safety and risk. These rhetorics are a major resource through which the GPs construct the boundary between general practice and lay therapy and problematise the practice of the non-medically qualified.

One way in which these rhetorics are employed is through the doctors highlighting potential dangers linked to the specific task of diagnosis. As such, they highlight their perceptions of the indirect adverse effects of the medicines. One doctor outlines what she sees as a crucial distinction between non-medical practice and the approach of the general practitioner:

I suppose one would resort to the medical model in that . . . I wouldn't miss serious pathology, that I wouldn't be treating someone with a homeopathic remedy who should be you know having their cancer removed sort of thing. I would say that's a safeguard for the patients in that respect that there is pathology that goes on which needs traditional medical and surgical treatment and erm, it may be that an un-medically qualified homeopath may miss symptoms which should be properly investigated.

(GP 21)

The extract below illustrates how such rhetorical construction is employed by some of the GPs with regard to their practice of acupuncture:

> I suspect that there's always the chance that, you know, someone'll have cancer that's causing their root problem and if the lay person's not very open to that there's always the possibility they'll delay a diagnosis or something where I kind of hope that we would, you know, have ruled that out or thought about it and considered it and everything before we start just drilling people with a course of acupuncture.
>
> (GP 11)

Some of the GPs refer to specific practice experiences and encounters with patients as evidence of what they perceive to be the potential and very real dangers of non-medical therapy. One doctor practising homeopathy explains his fears of lay therapists mislabelling complaints:

> what worries me a lot with the lay homeopathic person is, er, not getting the diagnosis right, you know a lot of, I suppose my medical knowledge is are you dealing with something serious? you know, if somebody comes to you with urinary symptoms or something like that am I treating this with homeopathy or has somebody got a bladder cancer? That's the worry on the lay side. I mean I've seen people who have come to me having had lay homeopathy and they've come to me with a set of symptoms, you know, for years and I've examined them and found serious illness. Now that worries me a lot. (GP 20)

In addition to the claim that lay diagnosis is dangerous and the contrasting portrayal of GP diagnosis as offering safety and protection to the patient, a number of doctors offer another presentation of risk associated with unconventional treatments. Some GPs explain lay therapy as involving direct adverse effects; that is, they highlight the 'direct physiological or physical impact from the intervention itself' upon the patient (Jonas 1996: 130). Here again, we have an appeal to the safety of a medical approach to the therapies, one where medical science and conventional procedures are perceived as *essential foundations* of good therapy. One doctor outlines a justification for his use of acupuncture in general practice:

> I think the safety of it, the safety of being medical and using something like needles, you know, there are a few points around where you are dicing with death, you can sort of puncture someone's lung if you put it in the wrong place and that sort of thing so there's the odd thing like that where I think my medical training and knowledge of anatomy and everything else like that is better.
>
> (GP 11)

And another GP similarly explains what she sees as the dangers of lay hypnotherapy:

> I think the non-medically qualifieds can do a lot of harm and they quite often do. They can implant post-hypnotic suggestions, you can suggest to someone that when they come out of a trance something might happen and usually it will or they behave in a certain way and they can implant ideas in people and they actually make them quite disturbed.
>
> (GP 16)

Rhetorics of scope: restrictive alternatives and expansive complementaries

> You can use [acupuncture] as an adjunct to all sorts of other therapies. What I mean is if I'm an acupuncturist solo, that's my job private outside, all I can do is treat people with acupuncture. Here I can practise, I can treat people with normal medicine . . . but I have this added, er, arrow in my quill which I can use for acupuncture.
>
> (GP 2)

To briefly return to the theme of diagnostics as found within the GPs' accounts, we can identify what is here termed the rhetorics of 'scope' and their importance in creating and maintaining the discursive boundary between medical and non-medical practice. The following extract from a GP practising hypnotherapy provides a clear example of the imagery of rigidity and inflexibility applied to the procedures of lay diagnostics: 'One of the things about lay people . . . is that doctors are trained from early on to have differential diagnoses and be prepared to change our diagnosis and lay people seem to be often very *fixed* in their ideas' (GP 5).

These rhetorical devices of flexibility and rigidity are equally employed with regard to the overall practice of the two different groups of practitioners. On the one hand, lay practice is described as characteristically 'rigid', 'closed' or 'narrow' while a pivotal defining feature of general practice is understood to be the GP's flexibility, rounded approach and awareness of possible alternative avenues to treatment.

Within many accounts there is a repeated use of the imagery of 'exclusive dependency' (GP 12) of the non-medically qualified upon single medicines: they are practising the therapies 'in solo' and they think their therapy 'is everything' (GP 22). This is expressed by some GPs in terms of a refusal by lay therapists to pass patients on to practitioners of other medicines even after a treatment has been ineffective:

a medical complementary therapist will say right this is an acute abdomen this will have to go into hospital, I'm not going to give it Belladonna. Whereas a lay practitioner might very well say well if Belladonna doesn't work I'll try another homeopathic remedy, you know whereas, I think you're safer seeing a medical person.

(GP 3)

This extract, like others outlined earlier, suggests a fear of the inability of non-medically qualified therapists to successfully diagnose certain conditions. In response, this GP claims that some lay practitioners may slavishly pursue their alternative line of treatment when serious illness may require the specialised intervention of other courses of treatment available only within hospital medicine.

Non-medically qualified therapists are described by the GPs as too adventurous in practice and as having too high expectations of their therapy's power to heal; an expectancy that in some cases is perceived as born of the therapists' dependency on one specialist therapy. The non-medically qualified are seen as 'heroic' in their approach, they are convinced of the omnipotent powers of their system of medicine and, as a result, often persist in treatment when this is clearly unsuitable. The following extract of talk of a GP practising homeopathy and acupuncture describes non-medically qualified homeopaths and their approach to homeopathy in these terms:

A lot of homeopaths think there's a remedy for every ill, you can cure everything, or every ill needs to have a remedy and it doesn't you know. People get ill and they get over their illness, the vast majority of them if they're healthy, have a good diet, they'll just get over it so you know every time you get a cold doesn't mean you've to rush off and get a homeopathic remedy, but a lot of the homeopaths are like that, all of but taking this remedy I wouldn't have got better, but you know a lot of illnesses are self-limiting and trivial and there's no point in taking a pill for every ill and that's one thing I don't like about them, the alternative therapists, you know, there's supposed to be a pill for every ill, you know, there shouldn't be a pill for every ill.

(GP 12)

As part of the presentation of general practice as a 'rounded' and 'flexible' style, some GPs also refer to a number of features of general practice (these include access to such things as X-rays, an array of different diagnostic tests, and the medical services of specialists in the case of referrals). These features are used to highlight the benefits of integrative practice and also to further distance general practice from non-medical therapy (the GPs stress how these features are not at the disposal of non-medical therapists).

The private sector of professional self-interest

> One's always cautious about private practice because, you know, especially when people are paying by the session . . . you wonder to what extent the financial angle influences therapy.
>
> (GP 18)

The private sector is condemned by most of the GPs as encouraging 'self-interest' on the part of the practitioner. These GPs suggest that non-medically qualified therapists are influenced by financial considerations as a result of their need to survive in a competitive free market. Indeed, some social science commentators have drawn upon this issue as a possible 'contradiction' or 'tension' facing lay therapists in their attempts to justify an altruistic approach to practice (Sharma 1992) and the doctors interviewed present a similar view.

This 'problem' of private practice is clearly contrasted to the motivation behind GPs' development of the therapies. As GP 17 explains:

> I'm not saying they're not skilled, I think some of them are very skilled but they take longer than they should for financial considerations. I don't know about the ethics of what they're doing. I do know about my ethics and my colleagues' ethics in the field who are doing it. I mean, I'm not doing it for financial gain. I do treat other doctors' patients when they refer to me but I don't take money for it and I will say if you really want to make a donation choose a charity that you can donate to.
>
> (GP 17)

The 'free service' of NHS general practice and the absence of financial considerations have been popular rhetorics employed by some sections of the medical profession to help highlight an altruistic ideal for practice (Calnan 1988) and this rhetoric is also prominent in the GPs' accounts examined here. As GP 10 suggests, getting complementary medicine for free on the NHS may be an advantage associated with GP therapy: 'On the whole the patients think [complementary medicine's] wonderful because they, also this idea being wonderful, because they perceive them as a thing that you would usually have to pay for'.

Rhetoric of access

> I think the big thing is that it's the balance between what we can afford to provide and how much do we encourage people to seek out these things for themselves because they can be quite pricey you know, and if, so if you're well off it's not a problem but if you're not well off it is a problem.
>
> (GP 13)

It is still the case that the vast majority of unconventional therapy provided in Britain is outside the NHS and practised by non-medically qualified therapists in the private sector (Saks 1994; Dickinson 1996). One rhetorical construction in most accounts which links strongly with this rhetoric of access relates to the cost of private lay practice and equity of provision. One doctor stresses, 'If it's given by your doctor then it's free . . . I'm always a bit concerned about the overall cost to the patient' (GP 24). This represents another rhetorical tool with which the GPs demarcate a boundary between non-medical practice and that of the GP within the National Health Service, with many of the doctors suggesting that a main motivation for developing their practice of complementary therapies is the inability of many of their patients to afford private treatment. GP 22 uses this rhetorical device in her talk. She says:

> I think that a reason I'm doing it is because that I feel a lot of my patients can't afford private acupuncture and they wouldn't get acupuncture any other way. If it's £30 for half an hour a lot of my patients are on income support and they just couldn't do it.
>
> (GP 22)

While the growing range of patients now seeking complementary treatment is acknowledged (Dickinson 1996), one possible barrier to the use of CAM is the inability of patients to afford private unconventional treatment (Huggon and Trench 1992). It would seem that these GPs developing complementary therapies within their surgery are keen to capitalise on such claims in their attempt to highlight the benefits of NHS GP therapy over that of private non-medically qualified therapists.

Discussion

The analysis reveals how the doctors demarcate two contrasting styles of therapeutic practice – complementary and alternative – in their attempt to distance GP therapy from non-medical therapy. Furthermore, building upon this boundary-construction, a significant proportion of the doctors' talk is directed towards attacking and undermining those classified within the accounts as alternative therapists and their associated alternative practices. A range of rhetorical strategies are employed by the GP therapists (the rhetorics of scope, the rhetoric of access and the contrasting rhetorics of safety and risk amongst others) to accomplish such occupational demarcation and distancing.

GP therapist criticisms of non-medical therapy support Saks' interpretation that the incorporation of CAM by the medical profession is motivated, partly at least, by a defensive strategy based upon self-interest (Saks 1995).

To claim superiority for complementary over alternative-style practice and to undermine non-medical therapy as dangerous and so on helps to claim a direct and central role for general practitioners in legitimate unconventional therapy. These presentations can be interpreted as attempts to promote the exclusive authority of the medically qualified over the practice of CAM.

However, the analysis presented here extends beyond Saks' work. Attention is directed away from the pronouncements of the medical elite to an exploration of direct integration via the analysis of the accounts of grass-roots GPs. Saks' work implicitly draws upon notions of boundaries to examine and understand the changing relationship between the medical profession and those therapists of alternative medicines located outside the medical community (Saks 1995). Yet, such work does not conceive of either the medical/non-medical boundary or the monopolistic strategy of the medical profession in relation to CAM as ongoing everyday practical problems for grass-roots doctors. In contrast, the present study helps provide a snapshot of rank and file doctors' ongoing demarcation between themselves and lay therapists and their practices.

Such occupational demarcation is particularly interesting on two counts. First, it aids the capture of CAM (currently an attraction for an increasing number of patients) from other practitioners more traditionally associated with these medicines by the general practice setting. Indeed, GPs' potential to influence ongoing debate about where and how CAM should be practised is highlighted when we consider the relationship between GPs and a large number of the patient population. The orthodox healthcare provider has been overlooked as one of the more popular sources of information on CAM for patients (Kohn 1999). However, general practice is the main setting where expert and lay knowledge come into contact (Tovey and Adams 2001) and, given their 'gatekeeper' role (BMA 1993), general practitioners are well positioned to exert powerful influence over patient choice as to when and how unconventional treatments are to be employed (Botting and Cook 2000).

Second, the occupational demarcations identified in this study also help these GPs in their attempts to 'naturalise' CAM to general practice; distancing from 'alternative' therapists is good strategy for establishing and maintaining powerful and supportive partners in the world of general practice. The incorporation of CAM within general practice remains a controversial topic with many within the medical profession still seeing CAM as a direct challenge to their biomedical training (Saks 1995). In addition, there has been concern regarding the suitability of CAM (which is often seen as holistic and time-consuming) to the resource-strapped NHS environment (Peters 1994, 2000; Norris 2001) and also caution about the appropriateness of integrating therapies which are seen to lack a rigorous evidence-base (Kohn 1999).

While attempting to import fresh technologies and techniques into general practice, GP therapists must guard against being cast by others in general practice in the same light as non-medical therapists. They risk being viewed as defectors by others in their professional community. As analysis of the accounts reveals, one way in which GP therapists can protect against such criticism is to re-express unconventional therapy in a form distinct from that practised by the non-medically qualified and therefore as palatable to more traditionally orientated GPs.

This chapter has illustrated how GP therapists engage in boundary-work which attempts not only to adopt CAM but also to monopolise the practice of these other medicines. However, we must remain mindful of a number of features of boundary-work. First, while this chapter focuses upon the medical/non-medical demarcation found in the doctors' accounts, it should be remembered that boundary-work can also relate to rivalries and divisions *within* medicine. Indeed, analysis of other areas of the GPs' accounts reveals additional boundary-work (Adams 2000), with GP therapists demarcating themselves both from their hospital cousins and also from those seen as developing an evidence-based approach to general practice.

Second, closely related to the additional boundary-work noted above, we must also remember that boundary-construction is episodic and therefore often inconsistent. GP therapists provide contradictory presentations of themselves, their role and the nature of general practice depending upon the focus of their talk. While remaining mindful of the constraints of professional culture, change will always be possible as grass-roots GPs draw and redraw both the borders between themselves and other healthcare groups and the division of labour regarding CAM; boundaries are not fixed but tailored to the specific ideological task at hand (Gieryn 1983: 792).

Such inconsistencies should not be glossed over or deleted from the analysis of GPs' accounts. On the contrary, the ability of these GPs to draw upon divergent interpretative frameworks in their different episodes of boundary-construction highlights a major strategy whereby this professional group attempts to secure dominance over competing groups in the field of healthcare provision.

Given these features of boundary-construction, further research is needed to explore the boundary-work of other groups relating to CAM. An investigation of members' accounts from other subgroups within general practice (for example, those GPs opposed to CAM integration), other branches of the wider medical profession (for example, hospital consultants) and beyond (for example, non-medically qualified practitioners) would supplement the present analysis and help unravel the ongoing credibility contests between professional worlds which are attempting to locate and capture CAM as an authentic component of different branches of healthcare work.

References

Adams, J. (2000) 'General practitioners, complementary therapies and evidence-based medicine: the defence of clinical autonomy', *Complementary Therapies in Medicine* 8: 248–52.

Adams, J. and Tovey, P. (2000) 'Complementary medicine and primary care: towards a grass-roots focus', in P. Tovey (ed.) *Contemporary Primary Care: the challenge of Change*, Buckingham: Open University Press.

Adams, J. and Tovey, P. (2001) 'Nurses' use of professional distancing in the appropriation of CAM: a text analysis', *Complementary Therapies in Medicine* 9(3): 136–40.

Allen, D. (2000) 'Doing occupational demarcation: the "boundary-work" of nurse managers in a district general hospital', *Journal of Contemporary Ethnography* 29(3): 326–56.

Allen, D. (2001) 'Narrating nursing jurisdiction: "atrocity stories" and "boundary-work"', *Symbolic Interaction* 24(1): 75–103.

Atkinson, K. (1996) 'Alternative medicine: availability and quality of information for health authorities, GP fundholders and the public', Unpublished MSc Dissertation, Department of Information and Library Studies, University of Wales, Aberystwyth.

Berman, B., Singh, B., Hartnoll, S., Singh, B.K. and Reilly, D. (1999) 'Primary care physicians and complementary–alternative medicine: training, attitudes, and practice patterns', *Journal of the American Board of Family Practice* 11(4): 272–81.

Billig, M. (1991) *Ideology and Opinions: studies in rhetorical psychology*, London: Sage.

BMA (1993) *Complementary Medicine: new approaches to good practice*, Oxford: Oxford University Press.

Botting, A. and Cook, R. (2000) 'Complementary medicine: knowledge, use and attitudes of doctors', *Complementary Therapies in Medicine* 6: 41–7.

Calnan, M. (1988) 'Images of general practice: the perceptions of the doctor', *Social Science and Medicine* 27(6): 579–86.

Dew, K. (2000) 'Deviant insiders: medical acupuncturists in New Zealand', *Social Science and Medicine* 50(12): 1785–95.

Dickinson, P.S. (1996) 'The growth of complementary therapy: a consumer-led boom', in E. Ernst (ed.) *Complementary Medicine: an objective appraisal*, Oxford: Butterworth-Heinemann.

Easthope, G., Tranter B. and Gill, G. (2000) 'General practitioners' attitudes toward complementary therapies', *Social Science and Medicine* 51(10): 1555–61.

Ernst, E. (2000) 'Prevelance of use of complementary medicine: a systematic review', *Bulletin of the World Health Organisation* 78(2): 252–7.

Featherstone, C. and Forsyth, L. (1997) *Medical Marriage*, Forres, Scotland: Findshorn Press.

Gieryn, T.F. (1983) 'Boundary work in the professional ideology of scientists', *American Sociological Review* 48: 781–95.

Gieryn, T.F. (1995) 'Boundaries of science', in S. Jasanoff, G.E. Markle, J.C. Peterson and T. Pinch (eds) *The Handbook of Science and Technology Studies*, London: Sage.

Gieryn, T.F. (1999) *Cultural Boundaries of Science*, London: Chicago University Press.

Grant, M., Barney, R., Wagner, P., Moseley, G. and Dianati, R. (2000) 'Alternative pharmacotherapy. Patterns of patient use and family physician practice', *Journal of Family Practice* 49(10): 927–31.

Halfpenny, P. (1988) 'Talking of talking, writing of writing: some reflections on Gilbert and Mulkay's discourse analysis', *Social Studies of Science* 18: 169–82.

Hall, K. and Giles-Corti, B. (2000) 'Complementary therapies and the general practitioner. A survey of Perth GPs', *Australian Family Physician* 29(6): 602–6.

Henderson, L. (2000) 'The knowledge and use of alternative therapeutic techniques by social work practitioners', *Social Work in Health Care* 30(3): 55–71.

Honigsbaum, F. (1985) 'Reconstruction of general practice: failure or reform?', *British Medical Journal* 290: 823–6.

Huggon, T. and Trench, A. (1992) 'Brussels post 1992: protector or prosecutor?', in M. Saks (ed.) *Alternative Medicine in Britain*, Oxford: Clarendon Press.

Jonas, W. (1996) 'Safety in complementary medicine', in E. Ernst (ed.) *Complementary Medicine: an objective appraisal*, Oxford: Butterworth-Heinemann.

Joyce, C.R.B. (1994) 'Placebo and complementary medicine', *Lancet* 344: 1279–81.

Kerr, A., Cunningham-Burley, S. and Amos, A. (1997) 'The new genetics: professionals' discursive boundaries', *The Sociological Review* 45(2): 279–303.

Kohn, M. (1999) *Complementary Therapies in Cancer Care*, London: MacMillan Cancer Relief.

Lewith, G.T., Hyland, M. and Gray, S.F. (2001) 'Attitudes and use of complementary medicine among physicians in the United Kingdom', *Complementary Therapies in Medicine* 9(3): 167–72.

MacLennan, A., Wilson, D. and Taylor, A. (2002) 'The escalating cost and prevalence of alternative medicine', *Preventive Medicine* 35: 166–73.

McInlay, A. and Potter, J. (1987) 'Model discourse', *Social Studies of Science* 17: 443–63.

May, C. and Sirur, D. (1998) 'Art, science and placebo: incorporating homeopathy in general practice', *Sociology of Health and Illness* 20(2): 168–90.

Nicholls, P.A. (1988) *Homeopathy and the Medical Profession*, London: Croom Helm.

Norris, P. (2001) 'How "we" are different from "them": occupational boundary maintenance in the treatment of musculo-skeletal problems', *Sociology of Health and Illness* 23(1): 24–43.

Perkin, M., Pearcy, R.M. and Fraser J.S. (1994) 'A comparison of the attitudes shown by general practitioners, hospital doctors and medical students towards alternative medicine', *Journal of the Royal Society of Medicine* 87: 523–5.

Perry, R. and Dowrick, C.F. (2000) 'Complementary medicine and general practice: an urban perspective', *Complementary Therapies in Medicine* 8(2): 71–5.

Peters, D. (1994) 'Sharing responsibility for patient care', in S. Budd and U. Sharma (eds) *The Healing Bond: the patient–practitioner relationship and therapeutic responsibility*, London: Routledge.

Peters, D. (2000) 'From holism to integration: is there a future for complementary therapies in the NHS?', *Complementary Therapies in Nursing and Midwifery* 6: 59–60.

Pirotta, M., Cohen, M., Kotsirilos, V. and Farish, S.J. (2000) 'Complementary therapies: have they become accepted in general practice?', *Medical Journal of Australia* 172(3): 105–9.

Potter, J. (1996) *Representing Reality*, London: Sage.

Rankin-Box, D. (1997) 'Therapies in practice: a survey assessing nurses' use of complementary therapies', *Complementary Therapies in Nursing and Midwifery* 3(2): 92–9.

Saks, M. (1994) 'The alternatives to medicine', in J. Gabe, D. Keheller, and G. Williams (eds) *Challenging Medicine*, London: Routledge.

Saks, M. (1995) *Professions and the Public Interest*, London: Routledge.

Sarel, A., Borkan, J., Carasso, R.L., Bernstein, J. and Rozovsky, U. (1998) 'Attitudes of family physicians to alternative medicine', *Harefuah* 135(3): 101–4.

Schmidt, K., Jacobs, P.A. and Barton, A. (2002) 'Cross-cultural differences in GPs' attitudes towards complementary and alternative medicine: a survey comparing regions of the UK and Germany', *Complementary Therapies in Medicine* 10(3): 141–7.

Sharma, U. (1992) *Complementary Medicine Today: practitioners and patients*, London: Routledge.

Thomas, K., Nicholl, J. and Fall, M. (2001) 'Access to complementary medicine via general practice', *British Journal of General Practice* 51(462): 25–30.

Thomas, K., Fall, M., Parry, G. and Nicholl, J. (1995) *National Survey of Access to Complementary Health Care via General Practice*, Sheffield: Medical Care Research Unit, University of Sheffield.

Tovey, P. and Adams, J. (2001) 'Primary care as intersecting social worlds', *Social Science and Medicine* 52: 695–706.

Vickers, A. (1993) *Complementary Medicine and Disability*, London: Chapman and Hall.

Vinker, S., Nakar, S., Amir, N., Lustman, A. and Weingarten, M. (2002) 'Family practitioners' knowledge and attitudes towards various fields of non-conventional medicine', *Harefuah* 141(10): 883–7.

Chapter 9

CAM and nursing

From advocacy to critical sociology

Jon Adams and Philip Tovey

Introduction

While the sociological analysis of CAM (complementary and alternative medicine) remains essentially under-developed, issues surrounding professional action and professionalisation have received perhaps as much, if not more, attention than many others (see Boon *et al.* Chapter 7). In this section of the book (Part II) we have seen evidence of this through discussion of philosophical boundaries, the professionalisation of CAM practitioners, and finally the appropriation of CAM by practitioners within orthodoxy. Indeed, when attention has been centred on orthodox professions, medicine, and in particular general practice, has tended to be the pivotal point of reference (Eastwood 2000; Pirotta *et al.* 2000; Adams 2001). This is perhaps surprising in view of the evidence that it is another profession – nursing – that is actually at the forefront of integration (House of Lords 2000). To date, writings on the interaction, or apparent affinity, between nursing and CAM have been mainly produced by advocates of that integration (Rankin-Box 1995). Consequently, the appropriateness of continuing integration is frequently presented as a taken-for-granted assumption (Tiran and Mack 2000; McCabe 2001) and potentially problematic issues (about, for instance, professional motivation and purpose) are avoided (Kuhn 1999). In this chapter we suggest a framework for subjecting the CAM–nursing relationship to a critical sociological analysis. We take the UK as our primary point of reference. However, the issues raised are likely to be of relevance – albeit in modified forms – throughout late modern societies.

In the UK, membership figures for the Complementary Therapies Forum of the Royal College of Nursing (RCN) give some indication of the extent of interest within the profession, and of the growth of that interest during the late 1990s. In 1997, membership (which is simply a reflection of interest and not of active practice) stood at 1,600; by 2000 this had risen to 11,400 (House of Lords 2000). Elsewhere, activities of parallel representative bodies in other advanced societies have mirrored this development (Royal College of Nursing Australia 1997; Fox-Young 1998).

This apparent growth, or cementing, of the affinity is happening more broadly at an interesting time in the development of nursing. There is an ongoing discussion of enhanced nursing roles. This is something, at least in part, that is reflected in UK government policy, as seen for instance in the evolution of nurse consultant positions, nurse prescribing and the centrality of nursing to the National Health Service (NHS) help-line: NHS direct. The potential encroachment into the traditional territories of medicine is inherent in these developments (Tovey and Adams 2001). Alongside these practical shifts has been continuing debate about the most appropriate form and content for the profession. Bound up in these debates are issues to do with the appropriateness of an aping of medical practice and, relatedly, matters of clinical and epistemological autonomy (Barton 1999). In short, the essence of nursing is frequently the source of contestation, and that debate is both played out through recourse to perceived historical reality and to the desired shape of future action (Watson 1998; Rinker 2000; Wilson 2000; Snyder and Linquist 2001). As will be seen later, reference to historical events is actively employed when these debates become manifest in relation to CAM.

This chapter sets out a framework through which this developing relationship between CAM and nursing can be studied. Explicit in our approach is the need to appropriately contextualise those analyses, notably in relation to the nature and location of nursing as a profession, to its historical development and its current structural and cultural position. Our approach is developmental: the framework has evolved from issues raised by our ongoing theoretical and empirical work on CAM nursing. It is a crystallisation of the many unanswered questions raised to date. Thus, before outlining the framework, we will summarise the conceptual and empirical context that has informed its production.

Conceptual background

Given the lack of theoretically informed work on CAM nursing, our initial task is to establish a set of sensitising concepts (Clarke 1990). The bulk of our conceptual apparatus is drawn from a single theoretical perspective – Social Worlds Theory (SWT). However, as our aim is to produce a practical and applied research direction for a sociology of CAM nursing, we limit discussion here to the most directly relevant dimensions of this perspective and direct readers to previous work for a more detailed and rich profile of SWT (Strauss 1982; Clarke 1990). We do not approach SWT uncritically. Indeed, as will be seen below, we introduce aspects from other theoretical work and programmes (boundary studies, the sociology of nostalgia and the sociology of stories) as a means of adapting SWT to the particular topic of CAM nursing.

A social world's framework is based on a conceptualisation of society as being made up of multiple social worlds, each of which is essentially interconnected and invariably predisposed to segmentation into smaller subworlds. Social worlds congregate around core activities or lines of work (in the context of this chapter, that of healthcare); they are 'universes of mutual response' (Shibutani 1955) in which members share ideologies about their activities and how they should be performed.

Worlds exist in many forms and are found in all spheres of life (Strauss 1982). Here we are particularly interested in focusing upon a number of worlds engaged in the arena of healthcare (including both professional worlds predominantly geared towards healthcare provision and production, and non-professional worlds more closely associated with the consumption of healthcare).

SWT promotes a conceptualisation of organised social life as being in a state of processual change: the key word here is *fluidity* (Tovey and Adams 2001). Worlds – through the actions of individual world members – are constantly shaping and reshaping their concerns, their territories and their borderlines. Likewise, they are forever participating in struggle and competition with other worlds (sometimes initiating division, other times forming new collaborations) in the attempt to capture resources, whether financial or otherwise. At the heart of such constant change and realignment we can identify a number of key concepts central to a social world perspective. For clarity, we shall outline these different concepts in terms of three wider groupings: concepts predominantly concerned with activities within a professional world (intra-world processes); concepts relating to the activities between professional worlds (inter-world processes); and those relating to the professional/non-professional world interface (status and participation of different world members and their interaction).

Intra-world processes

Fundamental to a world and its existence is its core membership. This can be relatively large or small, concentrated in a restricted locale or spatially scattered (Unruh 1980; Garrety 1997). While institutional buildings, practice settings and the like provide the physical basis to world activity, the very existence of a world is an ongoing interactional accomplishment by world members.

Social worlds are effectively 'universes of discourse' (Shibutani 1955), maintained by the rhetorical (representational) practices and actions of world members (Opie 2001; Tovey and Adams 2001). Plummer (1995) has brought world members' accounts further to the analytical fore with his sociology of stories. Following Plummer's lead, we can explore two inter-related lines of investigation. First, we can examine the 'social work [stories] perform in cultures' (Plummer 1995: 19) thereby positioning them more forcefully and prominently within the wider social order. Second, we can also analyse the role of social worlds in the production of stories: in effect, considering the contextual conditions (universe of discourse) in and through which stories are facilitated.

One particular process relating to world members' claims-making activities is *legitimacy*. This is the process whereby the value and worth of objects, technologies and members in a world are constantly evaluated and reevaluated; worlds are sustained through co-members repeatedly judging the legitimacy of different world components within interaction (Adams and Tovey 2000).

However, the landscape in which such assessment is played out is far from simplistic. Worlds are never homogeneous in their ideology, alliances and organisational structures, and the SWT concept of *segmentation* refers to the in-world divisions and groupings (sub-worlds) that invariably arise as different world players promote differing visions and directions for current and future world activity. At any given time there will be in-house tensions, fighting and negotiation about a number of issues affecting the world more generally. Sub-worlds are often the unit of focus for a social worlds perspective (analysing the processes that are geared towards establishing worth and validity within their world boundaries) and, as we outline later, this is a particularly pertinent concept for understanding and exploring issues relating to the development of CAM nursing.

SWT promotes an anti-determinist approach to collective action (Strauss 1982) and at all times members maintain the potential to create new meanings and introduce new practices and technologies to their world. The future of such new practices and technologies (while some become firmly established over time, others may disappear as soon as they are introduced) depends very much upon the nature and success of the accompanying *authentication* process. This is the process whereby entrepreneurial sub-world members attempt to naturalise their 'exotic' practices, locate them firmly within the make-up of the existing world and thereby counteract opposition to, and criticism of, their entrepreneurial behaviour. If members, and their activities, are seen by co-members as overstepping the mark then the threat of isolation or even excommunication is ever real (Strauss 1982). As we will see below, this is a pertinent set of conceptual tools for exploring nursing and the way in which the processes of integrating CAM are managed and influenced within world boundaries. Nurses adopting and supporting CAM are deeply engaged in authentication processes. It would seem that CAM nursing has developed its own 'ideological weapons' (Strauss 1982) in the attempt to secure CAM within general nursing practice.

Inter-world processes

So far we have outlined a number of concepts that focus primarily upon the processes within a single world. Yet, as explained earlier, worlds never exist in isolation but jostle and compete for resources alongside other worlds within an arena. As such, an important area for attention is the changing relationship *between* worlds. In this section, we outline a number of processes and features prominent when two professional worlds (of healthcare provision) meet and interact.

A major activity for any world is establishing and maintaining borders between itself and other worlds (Clarke 1990). This is closely linked to the world members' ongoing legitimacy claims. By claiming worth and value for a certain range of objects (animate and inanimate), world members also implicitly categorise other objects as of less or no worth and thereby exclude them from within the boundaries of their world. Drawing upon the supplementary boundary studies work of Gieryn (1983, 1999), we can see that world boundaries are not prefixed nor are simply the analytical problem of sociologists or philosophers. They are a problem for world members 'routinely accomplished in practical, everyday settings' (Gieryn 1983: 781) and also through more mediated communication (for example journal articles) (Unruh 1980).

While boundary-construction often involves the delineation of insiders and outsiders, we should not forget that arenas contain overlapping and intersecting worlds. *Intersection* is a concept originating from within early SWT (Bucher and Strauss 1961; Bucher 1962), and later revised by other researchers (Kling and Gerson 1978), that helps us to understand these overlaps and activities between worlds. In short, there is *strong intersection* where worlds not only share a concern for similar territory but also build alliances, networks and collaborative ties in order to make a new sub-world possible. In contrast, *weak intersection* refers to circumstances where a world may well expand and trespass into the domain of a neighbouring world but, in essence, adopts a technology or practice with no invitation to collaborate.

Types of world membership and participation: the professional/ non-professional world interface

While the SWT discussion above relates to *all* social worlds to a varying degree, we have so far tailored our outline of inter-world concepts to the investigation of meetings between professional worlds. However, worlds such as professional nursing, providing services and technologies, will interact with the user of their goods and services – in this particular case, the patient, their family and immediate social network. It is useful to explore a number of key concepts that may help us to contextualise and understand such professional/non-professional interaction.

Effectively, we can view the professional/non-professional world interface as a meeting of actors with differing levels of involvement and periods of commitment to the professional world in question. Such interaction can be viewed in terms of the world status and influence of the different actors involved. Here we can draw upon the work of Unruh (1980), which has provided a detailed review of various forms of social world involvement and participation.

Earlier we discussed the activities and existence of worlds in strictly monolithic terms, referring to one blanket group called world members. However, the positioning, status and involvement of those found in a world can vary considerably between individuals and across time, a point relating as much to non-professional visitors as to different professional members.

Unruh outlines four social types of involvement that characterise partici-pation in a social world: *strangers*, *tourists*, *regulars* and *insiders* (Unruh 1980). While not denying the importance of all these four types, for our purposes here, we will concentrate upon *tourists* and *regulars*.

Unruh defines tourists as those who 'have little, if any, long standing commitment . . . [and a] transitory relationship . . . to the on-goings of specific social worlds' (1980: 281). He describes regulars as 'habitual parti-cipants who are integrated into the social world's on-going activities . . . [and] have a significant degree of commitment to their social world through good times and bad' (Unruh 1980: 282). Taking these two social types as our starting point (and following a social world emphasis upon process, emergence and anti-determinism), we can begin to categorise nurses and patients in terms of the continuity of their involvement with and support for the social world of nursing. In essence, professional nurses can be seen as regulars and patients as tourists. Of course, these two categories – regulars and tourists – as they relate to professionals and patients are ideal types and as such there is potentially much room for variations between the two. Similarly, as will be seen later, with changing contexts CAM nurses themselves can become tourists, as they engage with user-based worlds.

Linked to these different levels of world participation are differing power structures that constrain and help shape interaction. Regulars, particularly those close to the core of their world, have not only familiarity of procedure and knowledge but frequently legal backing. These are resources often not available to more transient members and visitors and, as a consequence, the power relation between professional and non-professional is often unequal in terms of shaping care and treatment decision-making.

Power is a concept not readily discussed within the SWT tradition. Early work in social worlds, following the symbolic interactionist school of thought more generally, has tended to concentrate upon negotiation as the dominant process governing social life. However, power has more recently been made explicit within a social world perspective with the acknowledgment of inequalities in resource ownership and status both between worlds and different world members (Tovey and Adams 2001), and we have set out to adapt this concept further here.

Empirical background

As noted above, we have begun to integrate these conceptual underpinnings into empirical work on CAM nursing. Here we will briefly highlight some of the key themes that have emerged from one specific project. As exploratory (and indeed as yet incomplete) work, its significance lies as much in the leads it offers into future projects as for the results offered in themselves. Other empirical work that we are developing – projects still in their early stages – will be referred to later.[1]

The project to be discussed here was a text analysis of papers published in four nursing journals – *Complementary Therapies in Nursing and Midwifery*, *Journal of Advanced Nursing*, *Nursing Standard* and *Nursing Times* – between January 1995 and November 2000, by authors from within the nursing community on the subject of CAM integration. Given that advocates have been writing in large numbers on the subject, these unsolicited accounts provide a valuable starting resource for a fledgling area of study. We conducted a thematic analysis of eighty papers, selected by following tight inclusion criteria geared towards papers dealing directly with integration (Tovey and Adams forthcoming).

This early work has drawn attention to processes that can, in keeping with our theoretical review, be broadly differentiated into three main areas: inter-professional issues; intra-professional issues; and professional/non-professional interaction issues. In keeping with the developmental nature of our work, these not only tie in with the earlier conceptual discussion but also, in turn, form the basis of the framework for future work.

Inter-professional issues

As with all groups of healthcare providers, nursing operates within a web of professional worlds (and is indeed further characterised by its segmentation into sub-worlds – see later discussion of intra-professional differentiation). This introduces action at the point of intersection between groups with frequently competing priorities and, indeed, with varying histories and capacities to affect or prevent change. While these encounters are, in practice, often multi-dimensional (for instance, nursing as an entity must necessarily be played out within a professional network including managers and policy-makers as well as practitioners), for analytical purposes it is useful to focus on some of the core professional encounters. Evidence from our preliminary work suggests that CAM, professional differentiation and the development of nursing are closely interrelated. And the relationship with medicine is pivotal.

The familiar notion of medical dominance was frequently called on within the rhetorics of the texts. What is presented as a medical opposition to CAM (nursing) is located within a broader sense of the historical role of medicine as acting as a constraining force on the development of nursing.

There was an evident priority to establish professional distance from medicine in a way that naturalises CAM to the nursing environment and incorporates conceptualisations of medicine that set up CAM practice and medical practice as fundamentally incompatible. The conceptualisation of medicine is explicitly contrasted with (CAM) nursing by drawing on the imagery of a profession wedded to technologically orientated and essentially reductionist approaches to treatment.

Thus nursing is being presented as distinct from medicine, both as a consequence of institutionalised power relations and, more positively, by virtue of fundamental philosophical differences. Advocates of CAM nursing pick up these themes when arguing that CAM can form part of a professional strategy of proactive agenda-setting rather than reaction to medical authority. Thus, the agenda of a CAM nursing sub-world and its presentations on medicine are fundamentally interconnected.

Intra-professional issues

As we move our focus purely to the world of nursing, we do so on the basis of an awareness of *internal* contestation. Counter to professional representation, nursing is not a homogeneous world strictly maintained through consensus and harmony. In contrast, nursing houses a vast array of competing sub-groups who gather around particular technologies and practices (for example CAM, evidence-based nursing), specific healthcare settings (for example palliative care nursing) and/or shared philosophies and approaches to nursing practice (for example holistic nursing).

Just as it is important to consider the inter-professional context within which CAM-nursing activities are played out, so too it is necessary to appreciate the significance of the professional terrain and climate *within* nursing as an immediate backdrop to CAM-nursing activities and debates. The survival of a particular line of work within nursing (such as CAM) will be determined, partly at least, by the success or failure of advocates within appropriate sub-worlds to convince others in nursing of the legitimacy of such practices. Our preliminary work illustrates some of the claims-making activities and rhetorical strategies through which CAM advocates attempt to convince other nursing sub-worlds of the legitimacy of CAM, and thereby authenticate their new practices within wider everyday nursing activity.

One way in which this was illustrated in the texts was through a recourse to history – what we term nostalgic and nostophobic referencing. This was evident in many guises, but perhaps most clearly through the discussion of Florence Nightingale. Nightingale is used both to underpin the conceptual affinity between nursing and CAM, and to provide a legitimacy to the case for ongoing incorporation. The presentation of Nightingale is such that the bases of her philosophy, and what are often taken to constitute the broad principles of CAM, are almost interchangeable.

This referencing is useful to CAM nurses because it both draws on a defining icon of nursing – one that has been used in the claims-making activities of other nurses (McCabe 2001) – and because it implicitly counters charges of fad and fashion that bedevil CAM as a whole. As with discussion of medicine, such referencing fits well with an agenda geared to an enhanced position for CAM nursing.

Professional/non-professional interaction: member status and participation

Clearly, just as an understanding of CAM nursing must occur within an appreciation of inter- and intra-professional issues, so it must also be located within an awareness of relationships with other actors and worlds – both in terms of CAM nurses acting as tourists in unfamiliar settings and in relation to the impact of other actors and worlds visiting the CAM nursing sub-world itself.

Both at the level of rhetoric and of practice, 'the patient' or 'the public' are central to such a context. Indeed, the texts studied in our research reveal an awareness of the importance of engaging with the 'needs' of this constituency. The centrality of client interests, the interconnectedness of pursuing CAM and exploring other means of 'doing one's best' for the patient were themes drawn on consistently. The survival or prosperity of the CAM nursing sub-world is hard to envisage in the prevailing competitive professional environment without the capacity to claim patient interest to be at the heart of the project.

The framework

Our preliminary empirical and theoretical work provides the starting point for the development of a programme of research in the sociology of CAM and nursing. We make no claims that the following is comprehensive: merely that the three broad areas are a useful way of delineating issues, and that questions/themes identified within each are some of the most immediately interesting.

Inter-professional issues: some immediate research priorities

From our research on CAM nursing texts we have seen that authors are keen both to establish professional distance from medicine, and to argue that CAM provides the basis for a shift in inter-professional relations, primarily with medicine. Clearly, this is just the start of an examination of the interrelationships between CAM, nursing and medicine. For instance, beyond the rhetorics, we need to understand how the appropriation of CAM is being played out at a grassroots level, how CAM fits into existing nursing–medicine relations, and how far it can, in practice, provide a lever for change. We need to move toward studies in which day-to-day interactions may be examined more closely, and processes of sub-world protection and expansion are made explicit.

Away from medicine there are, of course, many other inter-professional relationships that are relevant to the integration of CAM. For instance, the relationship between nursing (and nurses) and the range of non-orthodox practices and practitioners is a potentially interesting yet complex one. For, while on the one hand there is a clear basis for what might be seen as 'an alliance of the excluded', on the other hand there are sectional interests to protect. For both, establishing the authenticity of their own provision is likely to be pivotal to the long-term viability of their practice. The strategies of both groups may or may not be compatible and processes will very likely be played out in different ways, dependent upon local circumstance. We can only hypothesise about these without empirical work.

Much of the work on CAM nursing to date has been concerned with describing nurse attitudes in a way that is devoid of context. There is a need to move beyond this to consider the social production of these attitudes and the mediation of approaches and events. We need to take account of the location of action. The nature of nursing–CAM relationships will be influenced by whether they are being played out in the state sector, the private sector or the voluntary sector. Nurses and nursing will occupy a different position in each setting. And, finally, linked to this is the need to consider the health context of provision. For example, we may ask: to what extent will the operationalisation of CAM nursing in, say, oncology differ from that for medically unexplained symptoms in primary care? The exploration of integration at different points in the system will provide the opportunity for the influence of differing patterns of inter-professional relationships and expectations to be examined.

Intra-professional issues: some immediate research priorities

Thus far in our work we have identified how historical referencing acts as a powerful rhetorical resource in the authentication of CAM within nursing. More particularly, we can see that nostalgia and nostophobia are both being used as identifiable rhetorical strategies by advocates of CAM–nursing integration. On the one hand, the presentation of CAM alongside discussion of a romanticised nursing past is useful in helping to claim affinity between these marginalised practices and the core 'traditional' values of nursing more generally. On the other hand, and often supplementing this vision of a romanticised past, we also distinguish and contrast CAM practice from more recent nursing practice and philosophy which is seen as dehumanising and overly dependent upon technology (like the wider society in which it operates).

But we have as yet a limited understanding of these strategies. How are such processes operationalised? In which circumstances do they evolve? Are these the strategies of public figures alone? Are they meaningful at grassroots level? Are other strategies employed in different contexts? Are they influenced by locally specific intra-professional contestation? We must retain a sense of the persuasive purpose of such rhetorical strategies and explore their role in the shifting power relations between the sub-worlds of nursing.

Beyond this, we also need a rather more sophisticated appreciation of the *selection* of CAM made by nurses. Clearly, we are not dealing with a single relationship between CAM and nursing, but rather a set of relationships characterised by both strong and weak intersection. As previous research examining medical/CAM relations reveals, the legitimacy and acceptance of CAM within orthodox health professions varies across the range of 'other' medicines available (Tovey 1997). For instance, the emphasis in nursing on aromatherapy, reflexology and massage rather than, say, acupuncture and chiropractic is widely reported (Rankin-Box 1995). While these various levels of acceptance are no doubt partly shaped by the dynamics of CAM clinical reality (see next section), they are also significantly influenced by political nursing debate regarding what nursing is and should be, what will prove acceptable to others in the profession and how the individual CAM will fit aspects of a wider nursing agenda. Future research needs to explore the reasons why some CAM are more closely aligned to nursing than others and how CAM nurses justify and present such contingent legitimacy.

In addition to the affinity claims and strategies directed at the grassroots of the profession, nurses involved in CAM integration also need to convince colleagues within other sections and levels of the nursing community (for example nurse academics, nursing management, nursing elites) of the worth of their therapies. It will be interesting to see whether, and how, authentication strategies are geared to the perceived character of the audience being addressed.

Likewise, there is also further scope for research to examine the relationship between CAM nursing and other less-supportive sub-worlds within nursing boundaries. What counterclaims and criticisms do these other 'oppositional' groups make of CAM, and in what ways does their specific use of rhetorical strategy overlap or diverge from those employed by CAM nursing advocates? Only with a wider focus upon different perspectives within nursing can we begin to provide an outline of the location and role of CAM within contemporary nursing practice and debate.

Finally, we need to retain a sense that individual nurses themselves have identities forged through the life process as a whole. To explore this, studies are being developed in which the individual life trajectory of nurses (studied via life histories) takes centre stage (see Note 1). Amongst other things, such studies will address how nurses first get interested in and involved with CAM treatments, how CAM and nursing interweave through the different stages of a nurse's career and life path, and which worlds outside of their professional setting are instrumental to CAM development.

Professional/non-professional interaction: some immediate research priorities

One acknowledged strength of SWT is its inclusive research approach, encouraging the incorporation of a range of perspectives on any one area or issue (Clarke 1990). Following this design, it is important that, along-side the activities and rhetorics of professional healthcare worlds, we also examine the perspectives and roles of patients within the context of the clinical reality of CAM integrative practice. Patients and patient well-being are central to the CAM/nursing interface, at least at the level of rhetoric – something noted in the talk of other orthodox professionals integrating CAM (May and Sirur 1998).

In this final section we will limit ourselves to outlining some of the core patient and practice-orientated questions raised by CAM integration that could be answered by future sociological work. SWT, with its specific focus upon member status and types of world participation, is of particular use in guiding future work in this area. Here we can also draw upon both past sociological literature (exploring patient–health professional inter-action (Rimal 2001) and patient constructions of CAM (Pawluch *et al.* 2000)), as well as our work-in-progress (see Note 1).

While we acknowledge various mediated interactions where patients may come into contact with the nursing world, our focus here is upon the real-time interaction between nurses and patients (whether in primary care, a hospital, a hospice or other setting). The practice of CAM by nurses raises a vast number of interesting questions relating to the clinical reality of CAM integration and the role and participation of the patient.

The clinical reality of CAM-nursing is affected by some of the constraints that impact more broadly on integration: workload (Greenglass *et al.* 2001), the suitability of state-funded healthcare systems for promoting CAM practice (Sharma 1992; Peters 2000) and so on. Thus, there is a need to explore the extent to which time and other limited resources constrain CAM integration. It may be, for instance, that some forms of CAM prove too time consuming, or that therapies require modification with nurses producing a style of CAM more readily suited to the busy work-world of nursing (a process identified with GP–CAM integration (May and Sirur 1998; Adams 2001)). Conversely, it may be that CAM practice is timesaving and thereby cost effective in some circumstances. For example, CAM treatments administered by nurses may help to calm and relax patients after major surgery and thus potentially leading to earlier hospital discharge.

All these clinical reality issues have an important bearing upon the patient's experience of CAM within nursing. Moreover, in the sense that they may influence the style of CAM practised by nurses, they have major significance for the conceptualisation of the patient within this CAM treatment setting (see Hughes, Chapter 2 for further discussion). Examination of the day-to-day application of CAM by nurses will provide us with the opportunity to explore the degree to which CAM nursing promotes the empowerment of the patient in both treatment choice and CAM specific decision-making processes and, extending our gaze beyond the confines of the strict healthcare setting, we can also analyse the role and influence of family, friends and other informal carers and networks upon the decision-making processes surrounding nursing and CAM.

Whether CAM nursing practice is challenging and recasting the patient–nurse relationship or is simply replicating more traditional practice dynamics between nurse and patient remains to be explored. There is certainly much potential for CAM integration to tip the balance of power between professionals and non-professionals. There have been signs that some within the nursing world see themselves as being in partnership with patients – a rhetoric in keeping with broader UK health policy. CAM is frequently presented as central to this partnership.

However, it is when patients actually take a lead role in treatment decisions that the potentially most interesting research environments are established. For here we can extend analysis beyond nurse-centred arenas. Concepts relating to types of world participation and member states are useful in such settings. In these sites we can explore the extent to which the (claimed) expert status of nursing is challenged, and the way in which roles as tourists and regulars may be redefined.

An example of the interconnectedness of CAM nursing with non-professional worlds can be found in a study currently being conducted by one of the authors, Tovey (see Note 1). The study concerns the mediation of CAM in cancer user groups. In this case, CAM nurses/nursing enter the arena as tourists and the issues that will be studied will reflect that peripheral status. For instance, one issue to be addressed in the work is how decision-making is undertaken about the use of CAM and the validity of various therapies and providers. The influence of professional worlds will be fully explored in this regard. It will be interesting to see how the rhetoric of patient centredness is played out alongside the professional interests of nurses as potential CAM practitioners themselves. Further, the study will provide the opportunity to unpack one of the core concepts of SWT – legitimacy. We can hypothesise that in such settings the legitimacy of actors, and the consequent legitimacy of their input, will take various forms and will have varying influence depending on issue. We might also postulate that the sources of legitimacy available to nurses may rarely, if ever, be the most powerful. For example, the legitimacy of authentic experience (of group regulars) or the legitimacy of dominant expertise (oncologists) may well occupy that status. Considering whether and how CAM nurses seek to carve out a niche in such circumstances will greatly enhance our understanding of grassroots processes of CAM nursing.

Conclusion

The lack of attention to nursing within the sociology of CAM has allowed CAM nursing advocates more or less free rein both to set the agenda of what is worth talking about and to imbue those discussions with a set of normative judgements that are rarely subject to critique. Thus the appropriateness of continuing integration is in general assumed, and central rhetorics – such as the centrality of patient interest – remain unchallenged. Elsewhere in the sociology of CAM (notably in relation to general practitioners), issues of power, status and professional motivations have informed discussions. However, despite the presence of anecdotal as well as some quantitative data pointing to substantial grassroots developments in CAM nursing, we have little or no critical analyses either of the nature of these developments or of how such developments might make sense within a broader context – a context informed by concerns of professional status and aspiration.

It was this prevailing lack of attention to the subject area that formed the background to this chapter and necessarily informed our objectives for it. First, our intention was to draw attention to this existing omission and, relatedly, to focus on the need for a critical approach to be applied. Second, we wanted to present a preliminary framework around which an initial sociology of CAM nursing might be constructed: one that was able to accommodate both a sense of the evolving nature of CAM nursing, and a recognition that actions will only make sense with an understanding of the place of other actors and of their interests in the process. And finally, we wanted to highlight how the themes and questions at the heart of the framework have been informed by our initial and ongoing empirical and theoretical work in the area.

Thus, at the centre of our approach is the need to couple critique with a full sense of the social location, and dynamic character, of CAM nursing. We have argued that the tools offered by SWT is one way, but by no means the only one, in which this can be achieved. CAM nursing as an entity will be constituted in practice, and the form it takes will depend on circumstance and setting. The fluidity at the heart of SWT provides the means through which we can begin to achieve an understanding of how the CAM nursing sub-world is emerging and why that should be so. It also fits comfortably with an approach geared towards an anticipation of division and sub-division, of contestation, claim and counter-claim. It puts a questioning of the assumptions of advocates at the core of work.

Our framework builds on such conceptual starting points to explicitly locate the CAM nursing sub-world at the intersection of inter-professional, intra-professional as well as professional–lay relations. As a result, our argument is not simply that understanding will depend on an awareness of, or attention to, context (as an abstract), but more that it will require us to consider the transactional dynamics operating between participants. When proceeding with the empirical studies – in which CAM nurses and nursing are central, or in which their involvement is transitory (as tourists) – that will form the basis of a coherent sociology of CAM nursing, there is a need to combine a sense of the interconnectedness of players with the critical distance that has hitherto been lacking.

Note

1 At the time of writing, relevant studies in their early stages include: an Economic and Social Research Council funded project entitled 'The mediation of CAM in and by cancer user groups, health charities and informal networks in the UK and Pakistan' (Tovey et al.); a UK Department of Health funded project, 'CAM and the care of patients with cancer' (Tovey et al.); the role of nurses as 'tourists' will form part of this. 'CAM nurses' narratives' (Tovey and Manson); and a University of Newcastle (Australia) funded project entitled 'New South Wales nurses' descriptions and explanations of their complementary practice' (Adams). Contact authors of this chapter for further details: Tovey at p.a.tovey@leeds.ac.uk and Adams at jon.adams@newcastle.edu.au.

References

Adams, J. (2001) 'Direct integrative practice, time constraints and reactive strategy: an examination of GP therapists' perceptions of their complementary medicine', *Journal of Management in Medicine* 15(4): 312–22.

Adams, J. and Tovey, P. (2000) 'Complementary medicine and primary care: towards a grassroots focus', in Tovey, P. (ed.) *Contemporary Primary Care: the challenges of change*, Buckingham: Open University Press.

Barton, T.D. (1999) 'The nurse practitioner: redefining occupational boundaries?', *International Journal of Nursing Studies* 36(1): 57–63.

Bucher, R. (1962) 'Pathology: a study of social movements within a profession', *Social Problems* 10(1): 42–51.

Bucher, R. and Strauss, A. (1961) 'Professions in process', *American Journal of Sociology* 66: 325–34.

Clarke, A. (1990) 'A social worlds research adventure' in Cozzen, S. and Gieryn, T. (eds) *Theories of Science in Society*, Bloomington: Indiana University Press.

Eastwood, H. (2000) 'Complementary therapies: the appeal to general practitioners', *Medical Journal of Australia* 173: 95–8.

Fox-Young, S. (1998) 'Nurses and complementary therapies', *Australian Nursing Journal* 5(9): 29.

Garrety, K. (1997) 'Social worlds, actor-networks and controversy: the case of cholesterol, dietary fat and heart disease', *Social Studies of Science* 27(5): 727–273.

Gieryn, T. (1983) 'Boundary work in the professional ideology of scientists', *American Sociological Review* 48: 781–95.

Gieryn, T. (1999) *Cultural Boundaries of Science*, London: Chicago University Press.

Greenglass, E., Burke, R. and Fiksenbaum, L. (2001) 'Workload and burnout in nurses', *Journal of Community and Applied Social Psychology* 11(3): 211–15.

House of Lords (2000) *Complementary and Alternative Medicine*. House of Lords: London.

Kling, R. and Gerson, E. (1978) 'Patterns of segmentation and interaction in the computing world', *Symbolic Interaction* 1(2): 24–43.

Kuhn, M. (1999) *Complementary Therapies for Health Care Providers*, Baltimore: Lippincott Williams & Wilkins.

May, C. and Sirur, D. (1998) 'Art, science and placebo: incorporating homeopathy in general practice', *Sociology of Health and Illness* 20(2): 168–90.

McCabe, P. (ed.) (2001) *Complementary Therapies in Nursing and Midwifery: from vision to practice*, Melbourne: Ausmed.

Opie, A. (2001) 'Thinking teams, thinking clients: issues of discourse and representation in the work of healthcare teams', *Sociology of Health and Illness* 19(3): 259–80.

Pawluch, D., Cain, R. and Gillet, J. (2000) 'Lay constructions of HIV and complementary therapy use', *Social Science and Medicine* 51(2): 251–64.

Peters, D. (2000) 'From holism to integration: is there a future for complementary therapies in the NHS?', *Complementary Therapies in Nursing and Midwifery* 6: 59–60.

Pirotta, M., Cohen, M. M., Kotsirilos, V. and Farish, S. J. (2000) 'Complementary therapies: have they become accepted in general practice?', *Medical Journal of Australia* 172: 105–9.

Plummer, K. (1995) *Telling Sexual Stories*, London: Routledge.

Rankin-Box, D. (ed.) (1995) *The Nurses Handbook of Complementary Therapies*, Edinburgh: Churchill.

Rimal, R. N. (2001) 'Analysing the physician–patient interaction: an overview of six methods and future research direction', *Health Communication* 13(1): 89–99.

Rinker, S. (2000) 'The real challenge: lessons from obstetric nursing history', *Journal of Obstetric, Gyneocologic and Neonatal Nursing* 29(1): 100–6.

Royal College of Nursing Australia (1997) *Position Statement, Complementary Therapies in Nursing,* Canberra: RCNA.

Sharma, U. (1992) *Complementary Medicine Today: Practitioners and Patients,* London: Routledge.

Shibutani, T. (1955) 'Reference groups as perspectives', *American Journal of Sociology* 60: 562–8.

Snyder, M. and Linquist, R. (2001) 'Issues in complementary therapies: how we got to where we are', *Online Journal of Issues in Nursing* 6(2): manuscript number 1.

Strauss, A. (1982) 'Social worlds and legitimation processes', *Studies in Symbolic Interaction* 4: 125–39.

Tiran, D. and Mack, S. (eds) (2000) *Complementary Therapies for Pregnancy and Childbirth,* Edinburgh: Bailliere Tindall.

Tovey, P. (1997) 'Contingent legitimacy', *Social Science and Medicine* 45: 1129–34.

Tovey, P. and Adams J. (2001) 'Primary care as intersecting social worlds', *Social Science and Medicine* 52: 695–706.

Tovey, P. and Adams, J. (2003) 'Nostalgic and nostophobic referencing and the authentication of nurses' use of complementary therapies', *Social Science and Medicine* 56: 1469–80.

Unruh, D. (1980) 'The nature of social worlds', *Pacific Sociological Review* 23: 271–96.

Watson, J. (1998) 'Florence Nightingale and the enduring legacy of transpersonal human caring', *Journal of Holistic Nursing* 16(2): 292–4.

Wilson, H. (2000) 'The end of Florence Nightingale', *American Journal of Nursing* 100(7): 24.

Postscript

Philip Tovey, Gary Easthope and Jon Adams

We introduced this volume by noting both our aim of bringing together sociologically informed work on CAM and by arguing that such research can be defined by its pursuit of rounded, fully contextualised analyses that stand in contrast to the frequently superficial treatments engendered by the quest for answers to practical questions. The contributions in this book have underlined how an understanding of CAM requires more than an understanding of specific therapies or medications, their 'objectively' measured character or their efficacy. It also requires more than seeing CAM solely in its relation to orthodox medicine. Instead, an understanding is required of CAM as a social phenomenon, subject to social forces which are historically contingent. We also need to see both CAM therapists and orthodox practitioners as active agents, creating the social world of a health care system.

We have distinguished three main areas to examine in order that an understanding of this dynamic can be achieved: consumption in cultural context; the structural context of the state and the market; and, finally, boundary contestation in the workplace. It is only through understanding these three areas, we claim, that an understanding of the development of CAM can be achieved. We argue, further, that these areas show both geographical and temporal variation. Finally, we contend that a full understanding of CAM's development requires an understanding of the intersection of these areas. Here, we briefly summarise how our understanding of these areas and their intersection has been facilitated by the book chapters, before setting out what we consider to be the implications of that understanding for future sociological research on CAM.

An appreciation of the active role of the consumer informs a number of book's chapters. For Goldner's respondents in the USA, choice is a commitment that drives them to mobilise as individuals in support of CAM – creating a fluid social movement. In Hughes' analysis, the link between consumer action and rhetorics of responsibility was explored. The push from consumers is also part of Dew's explanation for the success of chiropractic's case before a Royal Commission in New Zealand.

The increasing power of the consumer is matched by the declining willingness of the state to regulate both medical traditions directly. Rather, regulation of both is now achieved, as Dew, and Willis and White illustrate, through protocols of which evidence-based medicine is a prime example. And, as Collyer demonstrates, both are also regulated and influenced by the market.

This is not to deny that the state still has considerable influence, as Boon and her colleagues demonstrate in their study of the professionalisation attempts of various CAM therapies in Canada. There, the precise wording of a state Act means acupuncture can only claim to be a modality not a profession, while homeopathy, contrary to all its traditions, has to demonstrate it can harm people in order to obtain professional status. The state is, however, not the only arena where therapeutic boundaries are negotiated. As Adams demonstrates for doctors, and Adams and Tovey for nurses, the place of CAM within orthodox medical practice is a site of considerable contestation.

It is the intersection of these three areas – consumption in cultural context, the structural context of the state and the market, and boundary contestation in the workplace – that provides us with a fuller understanding of the place of CAM (embracing the evermore high-profile notion of integrative practice) in health care systems. Both Coulter and Hughes provide an appreciation of the paradigms that underlie much of CAM and much of orthodox medicine: paradigms that appear incommensurable but which are at other levels of abstraction remarkably compatible. Hughes demonstrates how, at the level of practice, co-operation if not integration is achieved. Collyer shows that, in the marketplace, both orthodox medicine and CAM are being controlled by the same company directors.

What this means for CAM research is that CAM must be understood with reference to its social location. Social location, in its turn, must be understood both historically and temporally. Any research on CAM must take into account international social processes, state-level influences (both at the nation state and, in federal systems, at the local state level), markets (including international, national and small local markets) and professional 'turf wars', both intra- and inter-sectoral. It must also pay attention to the justifying rhetorics employed by advocates on all sides to legitimate their position, without mistaking such rhetorics for the reality of therapeutic practice.

This is a necessary task if the sociological study of CAM is to maintain and enhance its distinctive academic role – one that reaches beyond the pursuit of narrowly established and temporally and spatially limited policy solutions. It will require cross-national comparative work to tease out the strength of the local, the national and the international in the development of particular therapies and their relationship to the orthodox. It will also require sophisticated, theoretically grounded explanations of the relationship between values, practices, movements and organisations. In short, we should explicitly recognise that the time is now past in which 'CAM versus orthodox medicine' provided a framework of adequate depth to underpin analysis. As demonstrated by the contributions to this book, CAM sits at the intersection of historically contingent, internationally connected, yet locally produced and contested social forces. And it is that complexity that should be integral to future work.

Index